PRAISE FOR HEALED BY CANCER

"You don't have to have cancer to read this book, but if you do, it's a good place to start your healing journey. Indeed, for anyone wanting to consciously avoid getting cancer or any other disease, start by reading this book. Either way, you'll be a better person for it."
-Joan Melvin

"A courageous documentation of a woman's search for her authentic self under the guise of healing from cancer. As the author shares her thoughts, I realized that I am not alone in my own *crazy* thoughts and struggles with behaviours and compensations to gain love and acceptance within my own family, society, and friends. She shares some tips on what worked for her and why. After reading her book, I am again reminded that we cannot judge a book by its cover and a person by their compensating behaviours, because we are all just trying to survive. This book gives some tips on not only how to survive, but also how to thrive in life."
- Jannie Chow

HEALED

by Cancer

A Journey From Fear to Freedom

JAYKA DUNCAN

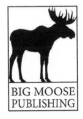

BIG MOOSE
PUBLISHING

To the loves of my life,
Ian, Jellina and John, you will always be in the sanctuary
of my heart.

Contents

INTRODUCTION
The Gift

Without knowing it, I had basically lived in a perpetual state of dis-ease most of my life. This particular state had been my norm for so many decades that I had forgotten what it felt like to live with ease. I was oblivious. Even when I was happy, my subconscious was still ill-at-ease. The undercurrent of my dis-eased existence was that of a low energetic vibration that festered mercilessly in my body for decades.

Cancer was my messenger of this state of dis-ease, and was essentially a gift. It was to be my choice whether or not I decided to unwrap this gift. Lucky for me, I was given two chances at it. The first time I received the gift of cancer was in May of 2007. At that time, I didn't even know that there was an option to unwrap this gift, never mind acquire the tool to unwrap it; therefore, the gift remained unopened. The second time I received the gift of cancer was in December of 2016. It took a while, but I eventually managed to discover the tool that would unwrap this gift.

This book is about the discovery and effective use of this tool - the tool of surrendering. Surrendering painstakingly unwrapped this infinite gift of cancer, layer by layer, until I had fully experienced post-traumatic growth and was presented with the ultimate gift of freedom.

Writing and publishing this book is one example of my dedication to surrendering. This book is so far out of my comfort zone it has made me feel quite vulnerable at times. The writing of it alone has made me squirm more than once. I am and will be sharing secrets that used to trigger shame. I'm showing people my inner world, a world that I had covered up so carefully. I will be baring my soul in a raw and real way throughout this book. Yes, there will likely be people who will shun me because of it, but I have to believe that there will also be people who will be inspired by me to do the same, and become more authentic themselves.

This book is about letting go of my image, this false identity that I'd put out in the world for so many years. It's a story that touches on every area of my life, at home and at work, in relationships, with money, sexually, mentally, emotionally, spiritually, and of course, physically. I want to share this story even though parts of it are deemed inappropriate by a good portion of society.

I can hear the questions already. "Why on earth would you want to hang your dirty laundry out for everyone to see? Are you crazy?" Considering the things that I will be writing about are all things I did and got away with without getting caught, I can definitely see the crazy in that. But here's the thing: I didn't really get away with it after all. As it turns out, I was my own worst judge in regard to some of my behaviours. As a result of my actions, feelings of self-judgment and shame festered in my body and created a cancer over the years. As my sister-in-law so aptly put, "Secrets will eat you up." She's right. You know what else will eat you up? Cancer.

I am able to tell this story now because I no longer identify with the woman who experienced those things. I have surrendered and released the guilt and shame, and cultivated self-love and self-worth in its place. I want to share my story to show how incredibly important self-allowance, self-forgiveness, and self-love really are. I mean, they healed me of metastatic cancer! If that was all they did, it would have been incredible. But learning to love myself and feeling worthy has gifted me so much more. And, considering that it's highly unlikely that I'm alone in this, that we've likely all done things that we're not proud of or have skeletons in our closets, this story may just create a-ha moments and potential healing for a few of you out there. Who knows?

This is my story of how I was healed by cancer.

PART 1

TRIAL AND ERROR

I call the first eighteen months of my journey with recurring breast cancer the trial and error phase. Yes, trial and error was the name of the game and unfortunately I was at the losing end of it. I was driven to heal my body and it was exhausting. Ironically, unbeknownst to me at the time, this driven state of doing was exactly what stood in the way of healing my body. I lived in a world of denial and was completely unaware that fear was the driving force of my life.

I had an intuitive knowing at that time that it would get worse before it would get better. And, it did. I found that's what happens when you put fear in the driver's seat.

CHAPTER 1

Getting The Diagnosis

December, 2016. I am sitting in the driver's seat of my car, by myself, in the parking lot. Crying. Screaming. Angrily banging my fist on the steering wheel. I am scared shitless! I feel my carefully designed precious little world crumbling around me.

What the hell had just happened?

Did it even happen?

Maybe it was all a dream, because it sure as hell felt surreal! Maybe I misinterpreted the whole situation. After all, I wasn't actually told anything. The doctor had just poked the crap out of me with a needle, without saying a word. But I sensed it. The writing was on the wall.

"Shit! What am I going to do now?"

I didn't want to think about it. I push down my fears, dry my tears, take a few deep gulps of air, and put the keys in the ignition. As the car starts, the radio comes on. Katy Perry's song, Hear Me Roar blasts out of the speakers. Well, if that isn't a sign from the Universe, I don't know what is! And yes, Universe, you're gonna hear me roar, goddamn it!

I look at the clock. 2:22 pm. These three consecutive numbers are my little sign that my favourite angel, my mom, is here with me. I feel her beautiful supportive love throughout the whole car. It actually makes me laugh through my tears! "Alright!" I say out loud, "I got this!" And off I go.

I make my way home. It is a drive that I'll never forget. From thoughts of "Bring it on! I've got tools now to deal with this shit!" to thoughts of "Oh my God. What if I can't? What if this is it?" to "I'm totally overreacting. Maybe I'm just worried for nothing." My inner world is turning into a gong show.

Somehow, I arrive home safely. It has been the longest three hour drive of my life. Somewhere down the highway, I made the decision not to tell my family about my fears. No sense in worrying them about it. "They did a biopsy," I'll tell them. "But it'll be nothing; it's just scar tissue. They're just making sure that's all it is."

Can you say 'denial'?

***

Well, this denial thing worked so well for me that a week later I showed up, by myself, at my family doctor's office to get the results. Feeling calm and confident that I had, in fact, overreacted, I watched the doctor come into the little room where I was waiting. She sat down and looked at me with a very serious expression.

"You have cancer."

I think the doctor continued talking. I saw her lips move anyway, but nothing more was registering. I sat there in a daze. My vision got blurry. My cheeks heated up as I felt anger bubbling to the surface. Tears were rolling down my cheeks. The doctor must have stopped talking as she was now sitting quietly, watching me while handing me a tissue box. I took one tissue and proceeded to throw the box across the room. It was uncharacteristic of me. It startled her. In a bit of an awkward fashion, the doctor got up. I could tell this wasn't easy for her either.

"I need to call my husband, Ian. Can I stay until he gets here?" I asked her, not wanting to be seen crying in the public waiting room.

"Of course, take as long as you need." she replied.

In between sobs, I managed to give Ian a couple of key words that had him bolting out of his office and at the medical clinic in record time.

I wasn't ready to go home to our kids just yet, so we went

for a drive. It was a quiet drive, each of us in our own tortuous thoughts. Looking out the window from the passenger seat of our car, I noticed that the world had just continued on as if nothing had changed.

We picked up some lunch at a drive-through as if it was just another ordinary day. Wanting something to distract me, I took a bite of my lunch. I chewed slowly and tried to swallow, but the food got stuck in my throat. I swallowed a couple more times. It hurt, but it finally went down. Food wasn't going to make this better, I guess.

Having no concept of time, we got back home to our two kids later in the day. Because Jellina and John had no school due to the Christmas break, they were both at home.

"I received some news today that'll likely shake things up a little in our family." is how I started one of the most difficult conversations of my life. "The cancer is back."

I could see all kinds of emotions come across our kids' faces. I stood up and suggested, "Let's have a group hug." The four of us hugged for a while when I made the next suggestion. "Let's scream. This will release some of our pent up emotions."

I think I was the only one who screamed. The sound that came out of my mouth was so guttural, so raw, that I sounded like an animal in agony. It was a horrific sound, and it scared the kids.

"Mom, please stop!" I heard John say.

There were tears once again flowing down my cheeks. My beautiful little family looked at me with so much love as they hugged me a little tighter. Through the agony, I could feel the gratitude of having them in my life. I was blessed.

Not wanting to ruin the Christmas season for our friends and extended family we chose to keep the news to ourselves and managed to get through Christmas, my birthday, and New Year's Eve under the pretence that everything was fine. Putting my expertise of 'pushing down those pesky emotions and covering them up with a smile' to the test, I gave a performance that was worthy of an Academy Award.

***

Any chance I had, I took my cute little therapy dog, Nico, out onto the trails where I would let my armour down a bit. This was the time that I would allow myself to feel the anger that I so often pushed down when around others. Angry thoughts such as "Really?! Have I not done everything in my power to prevent cancer from coming back? I've cut back on work; I eat healthy; I exercise. My relationship with dad is much better. I've taken loads of self-help courses...What gives already?!"

"What gives already?" would be the million dollar question whose answer eluded me for more than two years. What a journey of trial and error those two years proved to be. It was a journey of frustration, growth, despair, patience, forgiveness, anger, compassion, fear, learning about self-love and self-worth, and last, but definitely not least, surrender.

CHAPTER 2

Doing It My Way

Finally, we'd made it through the holiday season. January, 2017 arrived... a new year, and hopefully it would bring a new perspective. My brain fog had lifted a bit so it was time to buckle down and make some difficult choices. I had already made the decision that chemo would never be an option for me again... been there, done that. But I hadn't really figured out anything else beyond that.

A few more blood tests and scans were scheduled to check that the cancer wasn't anywhere else in my body. I also agreed to meet with the surgeon, even though I wasn't 100% sure that I would choose surgery.

The surgeon was a friendly young man who took some time to examine me and then informed me that I had the same type of cancer that I had ten years prior, and with it also being in the same location, he surmised that the tumour likely never left my body. It had just been dormant all these years, and eventually had grown about three times larger than it had originally been in 2007.

"How can that be?" was my immediate reaction. "I had surgery where the chunk that was taken out of my breast was at least five times larger than the size of the tumour. On top of that, I had chemo and radiation!" I was confused. "How can that be?"

"Well," he answered, "sometimes cancer cells can be so resilient that they dodge the surgery and survive all treatments. Those resilient cancer cells have multiplied in your breast over the past ten years and formed a tumour three times larger than before."

Wow! Are you kidding me? This was definitely something to consider.

We left the hospital with next week's appointment slip in hand which would be when we'd discuss other test results and possibly set a date for surgery.

"So, let me get this straight," I later said to Ian when we got into the car. "If this tumour now consists of a whole bunch of offspring of those resilient cells that survived ten years ago, then what makes the surgeon think that having surgery and chemo would be successful this time?"

As I pondered this, a quote came to mind by the brilliant Albert Einstein that goes something like this, "Doing the same thing over and over again and expecting a different result is the definition of insanity." Well, I might be a lot of things, but I'm not insane…at least not yet anyway!

With that in mind, along with meditating on it and weighing out the pros and cons, I came to the decision that I would not choose surgery at that time. I was willing to be open to changing my mind if needed in the future, but, in that moment it just didn't feel right for me.

With that decision made, off we went to the hospital a few days later for our second appointment. Let's just say that the vibe in the surgeon's office was not quite as pleasant this time around when I broke the news to him of my decision not to have surgery. I was so sure of this decision that I thankfully didn't buckle under the pressure that the surgeon laid on me. I'm sure he thought I'd fallen off my rocker or maybe that I had drank a little too much spiked eggnog over the holidays. But, the entire time that he was adamantly trying to convince me to have the surgery, using fear as ammunition, my thoughts were very conscious, overriding the fear. "This is just his limited point of view. All he knows is Western medicine. There are other options." These thoughts kept me strong in my conviction while exasperating the surgeon.

Over the following few months, I quickly realized that most of the Western medical staff were anything but supportive of my decision, making it painful to even get something as simple as a doctor's signature for insurance purposes. I felt like I had been red flagged. This is not to say that this is the case of all medical staff out there in the world of Western medicine. I'm sure that there are some that are open to alternative cancer healing methods. I just didn't have the pleasure of their company.

Having confidently scratched Western medicine off my list, now I had to decide what holistic method to choose. For those of you who have never typed "holistic cancer treatments" into Dr. Google, give it a try. Actually, what comes up is a maze of information on the ins and outs of probably a thousand different methods...from cutting-edge research of a variety of methods, to counter-research of these same methods, to success stories of this, that, or the other method, to an infinite amount of ads for supplements with huge claims. All of it was mind boggling and overwhelming to say the least.

What to do? What to choose? There were just too many options. It was quite overwhelming and I knew that I needed to remove myself from civilization and get grounded in nature to gain any clarity on the matter. My friend owns a rustic cabin near a lake in the Canadian Rockies where I stayed for a few adventurous days to see if I could figure things out. The plan was to go within, quiet my mind, and tap into my intuition.

It was February, with an average temperature of

approximately -20 degrees Celsius. There I was, in the cabin, trying to stay warm by a malfunctioning wood stove, having to go outside to use the outhouse, and relying on propane for lighting.

I had never used a wood stove before, but how hard could it be? To make a long story short, I ended up sleeping on the floor in front of the wood stove to stay warm, and also to stay under the thick blanket of smoke that was perpetually hanging in the air. No matter what I tried, I could not work the stove without smoking out the cabin! Turns out, as I found out a week later from my fire-chief friend who owns the cabin, the chimney had been completely plugged up and how sorry he was for that. It had been an adventure, that's for sure! I learned that you couldn't get too close to the stove or you'd melt your slippers, nor could you put your cup of tea on top of the stove, because it would explode. All in all, it was still a beautiful getaway where, despite the cold, the sun shone brightly every day. I hiked around the area breathing in the fresh air, in awe of the beauty that surrounded me, and allowed Mother Nature to calm my mind.

Refreshed and inspired to start my healing journey, I came back into civilization and made nutrition my first subject of research. I had always been quite a health conscious eater, but I wanted to kick it up a notch. I was already drinking green smoothies and juices every day. After reading up on the healing benefits of plant based alkaline foods, I decided to try a vegan diet.

I had learned that disease thrives in an acidic environment, so off to the health store I went to purchase pH strips. I had the option of peeing on the strips or spitting on them. While using saliva seemed a less awkward method, apparently it's not as accurate as a urine test. Every morning I peed on a strip before breakfast and again at lunch and dinner time. The magic number to attain was 7. Every day my numbers were as low as 3, indicating that my body was very acidic.

After a couple of months of eating a vegan alkaline diet, my pH levels did not budge. Feeling very frustrated about this and realizing that just the act of testing my pH was creating more anxiety for me, I quit testing.

Along with nutrition, I also researched holistic treatments and supplements. The sheer volume of information continued to be overwhelming not helped by the fact that people who wanted to help me, offered suggestions and sent information of different options for me to look at. Of course, I knew that they all meant well, but it tended to add more overwhelm to me than anything else.

I did, however, take the advice of one individual and contacted a lady who apparently was a gifted healer. She had success with several other people by helping them heal from cancer. I was excited, because not only did she live nearby, she also wouldn't take any money for her gift. Considering that I didn't have an income (and was fighting my insurance company), that was a welcoming bonus. It unfortunately ended up being too good to be true.

One area that I had been working on was to take charge of my own life, to trust my own intuition, and not assume that other people always knew more than me. My first, and only conversation with this gifted lady, consisted of her telling me that she would be willing to help me but that I had to stop everything that I was doing and only follow her protocol. In other words, she wanted me to hand over the reigns of my healing journey and let go of control. I won't lie, it was very tempting. After all, she was gifted; she was free; and, there were success stories that backed her up. Deep down, however, I knew that this would be a backwards step for me. There was the chance that I would possibly regress back to my old disempowering beliefs. I thanked her for her time and continued on my journey with me at the helm.

This didn't mean that I wasn't open to finding someone who was willing to educate me as well as suggest and discuss options with me. As a matter of fact, shortly after my conversation with the gifted healer, I learned of a holistic health coach, a lady who had healed herself of stage 4 cancer, fifteen years earlier. I decided to meet with her instead. She gave me lots to think about, along with providing some much needed clarity on the subject, and encouraged me to listen to my own intuition. Yay! She was speaking my language! I finally had something to sink my teeth into.

And boy, did I sink my teeth into it, in my usual, somewhat OCD, way. I chose a holistic doctor, had a bunch of tests done to figure out what the hell was going on in my body, and got the ball rolling.

CHAPTER 3

My Insane Schedule

The year 2017 ended up being what I call "the year of insanity". Although if you would have told me that while I was living it, I would have just shrugged my shoulders and smiled at you with a response such as, "I'm committed to healing my body!"

Boy, was I committed! A typical week for me consisted of driving 300 kilometres to the city on a Tuesday evening, staying at my brother's home overnight, and then driving to the clinic on Wednesday morning where I'd be hooked up to an IV for four hours, getting juiced up with vitamin C.

Once a month, I'd drive downtown to get blood samples taken, then I'd drive across the city to my colonic lady to get flushed out. I'd arrive back at my brother's home sometime around dinner time, and spend the night. The next day I would do it all over again except this time the IV pick of the day would either be Glutathione or Chelation. I'd once again drive across the city for my second colonic of the week. There were weeks that I'd also add in an acupuncture session or get something funky done such as cupping. Then, I'd drive the 300 km journey home, but not before fitting in a Costco run.

35000 kilometres were added to my car's odometer that year with me behind the wheel, and never once did I consider that this may be a sign that I was overdoing it just a wee bit.

For the rest of the week, while I was at home, I had a pretty regimented detox program consisting of 30 minutes on a vibration machine to activate the lymphatic fluid, 20 minutes of sweating in my sauna bed, followed by an enema and a shower. I would then spend hours in the kitchen preparing homemade healthy food, juice greens, and keep track of 37 different kinds of supplements. Next, I would continue to research different cancer protocols, meditate, take the dog for a walk, maybe fit in a nap, socialize with my friends and family, etc. I followed this action packed schedule every day that I was at home without fail.

I went for a check up at the cancer clinic every 6 months. As always, my nerves would be frazzled just by the thought of it. As the appointments came closer, my "what if" scenarios ruthlessly danced around my brain and my already sleep deprived nights were filled with even more wakeful hours. During the mornings of my appointments, with my heart in my throat and a jittery body, I would make my way to the cancer clinic for my ultrasound checkup. The radiologist would calmly move the scanner over the tumour, not saying a word while I was ready to explode with both fear and curiosity.

In July, 2017, I was told that there was possibly a 10% decrease of the tumour's size, but the radiologist couldn't be sure, explaining that he had to take human error into consideration. Therefore, it was essentially the same size as before by his estimation. "No change" was written on the report. I refused to hear the human error part of his explanation and clung to the idea that the tumour had indeed shrunk 10%. I was both relieved and disappointed by these results. On the one hand, thank god that it hadn't grown, but only by 10%, if that?

In December, 2017, I had an ultrasound appointment that went much the same way. Once again, my results showed a shrinkage of 10%, which was once again nulled by the doctor given the human error factor, and "no change" was documented on my file.

I had decided to start having infrared thermography tests done as well, but they also showed no change in my breast.

Really?! Ugh! After everything that I'd given up and everything that I'd done? Talk about frustration. "No change" just didn't cut it for me. The thought of "I guess I'd been a bit cocky when I believed I could have my body in tip-top shape within a year" was one of many that went through my mind. The other thoughts were more based around feeling I was letting my friends and family down. After all, they were rooting for me. What if I couldn't heal my body? What if I got it all wrong? Not to mention the "I told you so's" that I'd inevitably hear from the naysayers.

My inner world was in turmoil, but I kept most of these thoughts to myself and covered them up with a smile, because that was the game I played. "Nothing going on here!" The truth was my ego was hit pretty hard. I was feeling humbled and vulnerable. I felt the weight of the world on my shoulders and was getting pretty exhausted by it all.

Although I didn't realize it at the time, it was the beginning of a change in my perspective of this game called life. Up until that point, I had attacked my health crisis the only way I knew how - full force. I didn't realize then that the insane amount of effort that I put into this healing regime didn't just stress out and exhaust my body, but I was also doing it with an energy of desperation. Although I was oblivious then, I did eventually realize, much further down the road, that there would be no healing as long as my body was stressed, exhausted, and desperate.

September 16th, 2017 was a much needed, life-changing day. It was the day I participated in a San Pedro plant medicine ceremony in hopes that some light would be shed on the funk that I'd been in. I had participated in plant medicine ceremonies on numerous occasions in the past with amazing results, and I was ready to be inspired again. These ceremonies always gave me the gift of tapping into the wisdom of Source by having incredible chats with my higher self. This ceremony did not disappoint.

I remember it well. I was sitting on a log by a lake, surrounded by the beauty of the Rocky Mountains, when the initial message came through.

"Don't let cancer stop you from living your dreams."

This was the beginning of a beautiful, inspiring dialogue with my higher self in ceremony. "What do you mean?" was my reply.

"Start travelling the world, of course!" is what came through.

"But we can't afford it anymore! All of our savings have gone into paying for the medical treatments" was my instant comeback.

"Sell the house" was the simple reply.

"Sell my house? Really?" This was definitely not something that I had ever contemplated, and yet, the excitement that I felt rippling through my body was unmistakable. Sell our house...travel the world. That would definitely add some much needed excitement to my life.

"But what about all of our stuff?" was my next question, to

which the quick reply was "Sell that, too!"

Holy cow! I couldn't tell you how long I sat on that log by the lake, continuing to be in the company of my higher self, but I can tell you that I felt more excited than I had felt in a very long time.

When I came home, bubbling with excitement, I told Ian all about my ceremony and asked him if he was up to it. He replied, "Am I ready to travel the world, you ask? I've been waiting for almost thirty years for you to be ready!"

"Well, let's get packing!" I said. And, with that, we set our dream into motion.

The next five months proved to be even more insane than before, as well as a bit daunting, but there was excitement in the air! We were on a mission getting rid of 99% of our belongings...thirty years worth of stuff. Let me tell you, that's not an easy feat. We sold lots, gave away a bunch more, and the rest we either recycled or threw away. It was a detox in and of itself. All the while, we were balancing this with my demanding healing and travel schedule and Ian's full-time job. I'm not going to lie; it was a gong show. But, we did it. We officially reached the minimalist status by the end of the year, and were ready to leave Canada.

Before we left I had a few more tests done. Blood tests, urine tests, stool tests were all taken to see if my body had absorbed any of the supplements and intravenous concoctions I had been taking. When the reports came back, the holistic doctor sat me down and gave me the bad news. My body had not absorbed anything. Nothing. Nada. I had spent tens of thousands of dollars and it had literally gone down the toilet.

Fuck!

I remember asking the doctor, "How can that be?" The doctor had no answer other than that this sometimes happens. "I know you're a spiritual woman," he said. "I hope that you enjoy your travels and continue to meditate and find solace in that." This was the first time that I got the uncomfortable feeling that he didn't have high hopes for my mission to heal my body. I refused to give it much thought, however. Surely, I would be able to heal my body while traveling the world.

CHAPTER 4

The Game Changing News

The much awaited date had finally arrived. On February 6, 2018, after lots of goodbyes, a few of them tearful, we hopped on the plane, left the snow and freezing temperatures of Canada behind us, and were off to our first worldly destination.

Yelapa, Mexico is a quaint little fishing village off the coast of Puerto Vallarta where there isn't a highrise hotel to be found and the mode of transportation is often still by mule. We spent ten whole weeks with sand between our toes, breathing in fresh ocean air, and going to sleep to the sound of the surf crashing on the shore. How does it get any better than that? Considering we'd never had more than two or three weeks of consecutive vacation days, ten weeks seemed like forever!

We made weekly trips to a holistic medical clinic in Puerto Vallarta, which was just a 45 minute water taxi trip away. They offered IV treatments, but I needed to give that a break. For one, my veins were in terrible shape from all the needles. I had a lot of scar tissue that had built up and my veins were collapsing, making it painful and difficult to get a needle in anywhere. Along with that, in light of the test results I'd recently received, I was no longer convinced that it was going to heal my body.

I decided to meet with the American doctor that worked at the clinic to see what he recommended. This doctor had Western, Chinese, and Holistic medical degrees. The man was brilliant. My ears are still buzzing from that first meeting. Talk about information overload! One of the practices that he promoted to restore the nutrients in my body was urophagia, aka urine therapy, aka drinking your own urine. What? Could I even do that?

Believe it or not, I tried it. First, I drank lots of water so that the urine was diluted, then I collected the urine and, you guessed it, bottoms up!

Oh, the things I wouldn't do for a healthy body.

Okay, maybe I didn't exactly go 'bottoms up' with it. I took baby steps. First, I rubbed it on my lips. Surprisingly enough, it didn't taste that bad at all. Then, I put a drop on my tongue. Still, not too bad. Next, I took a teeny, tiny little sip. That's when my mind stepped in and said, "Whoa! Wait a minute. This is disgusting!" And that was the end of that little experiment.

Not wanting to totally give up on it, I decided to meditate on the question, "Will urine therapy heal my body from cancer?" Tapping into my intuition gave me the answer I was secretly hoping for. Drinking urine felt heavy in my body which told me that it, indeed, would not work. I scrapped that idea without hesitation.

In the end, I booked weekly colonics at the clinic to help me with my bowel movements. That was it. I had no other treatments. I decided to do a full 180 concerning my healing regime and stop the insanity. I finally started to realize that my body needed rest…a lot of rest. As a result, there were many lazy days, lounging in the hammock, wandering the beach, floating in the ocean, doing yoga, meditating, and making new friends. Surely, this is how my body could finally heal. It was all heavenly, and I was indeed feeling very relaxed. Would it be enough?

Our time in Mexico flew by and before I knew it, Ian left for Canada to help his ailing mum while I was getting ready for my next worldly destination - Europe. First stop was England for twelve days, then six weeks in France, followed by two weeks in my birthland, the Netherlands. I met some fantastic people, saw some incredible sights, visited with my wonderful Dutch relatives, took a couple of The Journey courses by Brandon Bays, and had ample time to relax.

All was well in my world, or was it?…Not quite.

While in the Netherlands, I started to experience some stabbing pain in my breast and armpit, something that I had not felt before. This scared the crap out of me. Could it be that the cancer had spread into my lymph nodes? Just the thought alone caused my throat to close up and a knot to form in my stomach. I was freaked out and told no one about it. With Ian in Canada during this time, I didn't want to tell him this over the phone. I also didn't want to worry any of my relatives. I kept it to myself.

At one point I was out walking by myself, feeling raw and emotional. It had just finished raining. As I was crossing a small bridge, I looked to the right and there was a gorgeous cloud with a silver lining. Then, I looked to the left and there was a beautiful rainbow. I just stood there and took it in. The universe was yet again showing its magic and the timing couldn't have been more perfect. When I got back to my cousin's home, I googled the spiritual meaning of both. This is what I found:

A cloud with a silver lining means that we should never feel hopeless because difficult times always lead to better days.

A rainbow is symbolic for the end of a transition, crisis, change, or upheaval, and is a sign of a breakthrough.

Well, if that didn't put a smile on my face and made me feel just a wee bit lighter.

Within a couple of weeks I was back in Canada and scheduled both a thermography and an ultrasound exam.

As the appointment dates drew nearer and nearer, my anxiety intensified more and more. I had myself convinced that the cancer had spread into the lymph nodes and that this was to be the end of me. I had more sleepless nights. Even my meditations didn't bring me the usual relief from the monkey mind.

As I sat waiting for the results of the thermography, I breathed deeply to calm my nervous system. I focused on positive thoughts. Thankfully, the thermography exam showed no change in the tumour, and also no cancer in the lymph nodes. At this point I didn't even care that the tumour hadn't shrunk. I was just so relieved that it hadn't spread into the lymph nodes. Hallelujah!

With that good news, I headed to the cancer clinic where I had my ultrasound exam. This time I was definitely in a better head space. As I sat there watching the radiologist do his thing, I asked if he was able to differentiate between scar tissue and the tumour. His answer was no.

What? Are you kidding? That was not the answer I was expecting. Knowing that I had a significant mass of scar tissue in my breast from the lumpectomy that I had in 2007, and also knowing that the tumour had intertwined itself within the scar tissue, his answer meant that these check ups had been a huge waste of my time and his. To think of all the anxiety that I'd felt leading up to these appointments, for nothing! Ugh.

Regardless, we spent five beautiful, outdoorsy weeks in

Canada that summer, both at a friend's cabin in the woods and on a campground, in a luxurious Taj Mahal camper that friends of ours lent to us. I was incredibly grateful for the generosity of our friends and family. I rested, we volunteered at our favourite music festival, and hung out with many friends and family.

At the end of August, Ian and I set off to Asia to continue our worldly travels with plans to spend at least six months there. Those six months ended up turning into eight-and-a-half months. If that wasn't an indication of how much we loved Asia, I don't know what is.

We took our time in each country, settling in every little village for a minimum of ten days, so that I had ample time to rest and meditate. Not being the city slicker types, we often would fly to a city and get out of Dodge as soon as possible, in search of jungles and beaches. The benefit of our prolonged stays were that we really got to know each area well and feel more at home with the locals. We fell in love with the locals no matter where we were. Not once were we treated poorly and I felt comfortable enough to venture out on my own on many occasions. I have no words to describe how incredibly beautiful Mother Nature is over there, and I can't remember how many times I had to pinch myself because I just felt so incredulous that I was lucky enough to spend several months in this magnificent corner of our world.

While in Asia, we visited Indonesia, Malaysia, India,

Thailand, and Vietnam. Each country had its own charm and its own reason for us to want to go back. At the beginning of our trip, life was wonderful. I felt incredibly grateful to be able to cruise around Asia, mostly on the back of a scooter. I was pretty much able to pretend that I had no worries, that there was no cancer in my body...that is until I received some heart-wrenching news towards the end of October, while we were in Malaysia.

The news that brought me to my knees was that the cancer had, in fact, metastasized to my cervix and uterus...fuck! I remember the moment I found out like it was yesterday. It felt like the world had stopped turning. I was light-headed and my whole body was vibrating. My greatest fear had come true. The cancer had actually spread. I now had tumours in three different places. Three out of four people die within five years when in this predicament. That just hit me like a ton of bricks. It was finally hitting home and I was no longer able to be in denial.

Holy shit!

Initially, when I was diagnosed with breast cancer almost two years earlier, I had a few additional tests done to make sure that there wasn't cancer elsewhere in my body. Sure enough, a red flag popped up on one of the tests. I received a call from the hospital back in February of 2017 that they wanted me to see a specialist regarding a growth in my reproductive area. I agreed to meet with this specialist to get his opinion on the prognosis; however, when I asked him about it, he said that the only way for him to be sure that it was benign was to perform a biopsy. By then, I had done a fair bit of research on the safety of biopsies and learned that this procedure actually damages the wall of the tumour which can significantly heighten the risk of the cancer spreading. When I brought this up with the doctor, he blew it off and told me that it was safe and that I had nothing to worry about.

By this time I had started to really question Western medicine and its role in the world of cancer. I was pretty infuriated at his lackadaisical response. I went home to think about it and made the conscious decision not to have the biopsy procedure done. If I was going to heal my body holistically, my reproductive area would be part of that whole as well. We decided not to tell anyone about the growth in my reproductive area so there wouldn't be even more fear projected towards us.

Here I was in Malaysia, about 18 months later, in total shock, and finally willing to admit that deep down I had known that things were not okay in my reproductive area. I had known that there was a high probability that the growth was, in fact, cancerous. Symptoms had been there. Symptoms don't lie.

I also knew that cervical cancer often doesn't show symptoms until the later stages and I had been experiencing them for a while. Despite being aware of all of this, I had not been willing to go there, not wanting to put any energy into it. Instead, I stuffed down my fears, covered them up with a smile, and continued on as if all was well.

Denial, denial, denial!

Well, no more! This life-changing, infuriating, devastating news forced me to come face-to-face with the knowledge that the cancer was in fact gaining ground. My game of pretending that everything was great had come to a screeching halt.

Now what?

I was at a complete loss. I was devastated. Why couldn't I freakin' heal my body already? What was I doing wrong? The desperation within me spread like wildfire. My heart was pounding and I was flailing out of control. "Other people are healing their bodies with less than what I've put myself through. Why couldn't I? It's not fair! What else do I need to do?" For the first time since I started the journey with cancer, I had no comeback. I didn't know what to do anymore. I felt raw, vulnerable, and so tired.

There I was, brought to my knees...

After spending nearly two years trying to make my body healthy, I felt a subtle shift starting to happen within me in that moment of being brought to my knees. There was almost a feeling of relief, an inner knowing, that arose within me. It was a knowing that I didn't have to go at this alone anymore. It was a knowing that I was ready to surrender. As a response to this knowing, I uttered the words "show me" in meditation.

I was finally able to get out of my own way and let my body become healthy. This is the point where my true healing journey began, almost two years after the diagnosis. It was to be a journey of surrendering, allowing myself to feel vulnerability, overriding the urge of denial, and discovering self-worth and self-love. In this state, being with my emotional pain body and dissolving it, I was finally able to uncover the core of my health crisis and ultimately bring the healing vibrancy back into my body. I feel called to share my story despite feeling somewhat vulnerable about the sharing of it. As a matter of fact, the writing of this book is part of my surrendering commitment. I am surrendering to love.

CHAPTER 5

Uncovering My Authentic Self

One of the many gifts I received of traveling around the world was to experience different cultures and how these cultures have influenced people's beliefs, thoughts, and ultimately their behaviour, including how they present themselves to each other and the world. Witnessing this made me more aware that no matter where we live, who we are, or what our status is, most of us want to fit in and be accepted by society.

It was no surprise to find that we are influenced by our culture and peers. I realized that I had been no different. I had created my identity in a way that reflected my culture. I had put incredible stress on my body, both emotionally and physically, and behaved in ways that I thought would make me be more worthy and lovable to society.

I also realized that who I was in Canada and who I became while traveling the world was not quite the same. When we returned to Canada after our travels, I started hanging out with friends and family who had known me for years. I started to go back to the behaviours and beliefs of the person who I used to be. It was subtle, but I felt it. This was partly because of the expectations that people had of me and the projections that they often unknowingly threw my way. But it also had to do with my own subconscious programming.

Elsewhere in the world, people didn't know me. I was able to be whomever I wanted to be. My commitment to surrendering my false egoic identity and reprogramming myself was definitely made easier while I was traveling around the world for exactly that reason. No one really had detailed beliefs or expectations of me, giving me free reign to be and allowing me to recreate myself and become a healthier version of me.

The challenge of maintaining the ground that I had gained while traveling became apparent pretty quickly. It would be easy to fall back into my old behavioural patterns, but I knew that the stakes were too high for me to do that. My old programming made me really sick and there was absolutely no way that I was willing to sabotage the healing journey that I continued to be on.

What did that mean? It meant that I had to go against my fear-based egoic reactions and be out of my comfort zone…a lot! I would do whatever it took to avoid falling back into those patterns even if it meant that I would be going against society's expectations. I was committed to being as authentic as possible. There would be no more hiding, no more dimming my light, and no more trying to fit into society. I had finally found the courage to be seen as my true self.

Don't get me wrong. I had to dig deep in order to find the courage to show up and have the willingness to be vulnerable. It wasn't necessarily easy to step out of that zone of society's expectations and dare to present myself in an authentic way with the focus on self-love.

Despite my willingness to be vulnerable, I would like to share a tool with you that if used effectively, will allow you to read my story while letting go of any judgments that you may have towards me, yourself, or anyone.

I learned this tool a few years ago from a beautiful and wise Indigenous elder in British Columbia, Canada. I was blessed enough to attend a retreat led by this elder where he enlightened us with the aboriginal teachings of the Medicine Wheel in concert with the plant medicines, Ayahuasca and Huashuma (aka San Juan). It was a powerful week. One of these teachings that stands out for me is based on the phrase "I am that too".

"I am that too" is an amazing tool that I've used countless times since being taught it at this retreat. These four little words can take us from judgment to compassion in a split second. It's powerful and it works. The beauty of it is so simple. "I am that too" is based on the fact that we've all been there, done that, if not in this lifetime, then surely in another.

I was able to put this teaching to good use within days of being home after this week-long retreat when I was sitting at an intersection watching a truck speed through a red light while the driver was talking on his cellphone. Thankfully, all the other drivers were paying attention and there were no collisions. As I sat there at this intersection in utter disgust, I felt all kinds of judgments for this truck driver. Then, I remembered the "I am that too" exercise and softly spoke the words out loud.

"I am that too."

Instantly, I felt the judgments disappear. Of course, I had driven distracted before. Although I tried to avoid it, there were times that I had answered phone calls, read texts, changed music channels, or ate a sandwich while behind the wheel. Who am I to judge this guy? With that, I had let go of my judgments and continued on with my drive, feeling light-hearted.

This was a far cry from the previous time that I had encountered a distracted driver, just a few weeks earlier, prior to being at the retreat. That time, I had been cut off by a middle aged woman and had narrowly escaped a collision. This woman had been completely oblivious of any wrongdoing because she had been too busy chatting away on her phone. I had such strong judgments of her, especially because I had literally just had the distracted driving chat with my sixteen year old son, who had passed his driver's test the previous day. I remember being so angry at this woman that I even wrote a post on Facebook about it, something along the lines of "How can we expect our kids to be safe drivers when there are irresponsible middle-aged people out there on our roads setting such poor examples!"

As you can imagine, I did not feel light-hearted at all. Instead, I kept the judgmental, angry vibe going for the entire day by thinking about it, talking about it, and discussing it on social media. In other words, I let it ruin my day.

The gist of this tool is that we have a choice in every moment of how we are going to react towards an individual, in a situation, or to a story (such as mine). We can be judgmental and angry, or we can allow ourselves to be able to relate to it somehow and feel compassion, understanding, and allowance. The latter are all emotions that have higher frequencies which will keep us feeling great throughout the day. Not only will the "I am that too" exercise help the people around us that we'd otherwise judge, it helps our inner vibration, too, by keeping the stress hormones at bay and making us feel more lighthearted instead. It's a win-win situation.

CHAPTER 6

Blissfully Unaware

I f you had asked me five, ten, twenty years ago how I'd rate my happiness on a scale of one to ten, I would have told you that I'd rate myself pretty high, at least an eight or nine. I considered myself a pretty happy-go-lucky gal, and felt grateful for the life that I had. Despite a couple of dark clouds that hovered around, I believed that I had a great life. I had a beautiful, loving husband and two amazing kids; I enjoyed my work most of the time; I had wonderful friends; I loved our family activities such as camping, sports, music, and lots of other stuff. The list goes on and on.

Was I faking it for all those years, then?

I realize now how much I had been fooling most people for years by covering everything up with a smile and embracing the attitude of "Nothing going on here!" That makes me seem pretty inauthentic, doesn't it? Not a very nice label to be stuck with, that's for sure. I'm guessing that my friends and family will probably feel a bit cheated by it too, when they realize what my game was. They may think they know me when in reality, all they got was my smiley performance.

The thing is, I really had no idea at the time that I was fooling people because I had fooled myself most of all. This performance was all I knew my life to be and all I knew how to be. I didn't know any better. I was blissfully unaware.

Approximately 95% of who we are is programmed in our subconscious. This programming is created by the experiences of our past, especially during childhood. Initially, we adopt a behaviour in order to feel safe, making it a survival technique. The problem is that as we get older, the threat that resulted in the creation of the technique in the first place is likely no longer there. Because we have been programmed in such a way that we don't know any better, we often continue in the same manner for the rest of our lives.

What were my programs? Here's one: doing whatever it took to avoid rocking the boat by being a people pleaser extraordinaire.

Here's another: sweeping all my stresses and problems under the rug pretending that they didn't exist. It worked brilliantly! It meant that I no longer needed to worry about anything and could live happily ever after… or at least that was the plan. This plan worked like a charm for decades.

So, why mess with a good thing? What's up with all the shit-disturbing shenanigans that I'd gotten myself into with surrendering to everything under the sun? I finally had that a-ha moment of how to get rid of that uninvited guest (cancer, of course), who'd been crashing my party for almost two years.

This solution would burst my ego-based happy-go-lucky bubble, but I was finally willing to let that happen. It took me long enough! And, it wasn't because there were no signs along the way, because there certainly were. Like that little nudge I got back in the winter of 2017…let me rephrase that…I probably got lots of nudges back then, but I actually became aware of this particular little nudge. It served me well at that time but apparently I was not ready to completely burst my comfort zone bubble just yet, so it was to be only a one-off. Better than nothing though, right? Here's what happened.

It was a month or so after getting the diagnosis. Ian had done or said something the previous day that had upset me enough that I had lost sleep over it. In the past I would have swept that under the rug; however this nudge made me realize that avoiding confrontation would not help the healing of my body, no matter how insignificant it may have seemed to be. It also created an awareness within me that I needed to come clean on a bigger scale.

We were on the road. Ian was driving while I was sitting

in the passenger seat with my brain going in overdrive. My body was overheating and my heart was pounding uncomfortably while I was navigating the inner conflict. Not wanting to do this but knowing I needed to, I finally gathered up the courage and asked Ian to pull into a deserted parking lot so that we could talk in the privacy of our car. I was a nervous wreck. I started our talk with "None of what I'm about to say is meant to hurt you. I have avoided confrontation all these years for that exact reason. I love you and I don't want to hurt you. However, I also know that I have to break this habit if I want to heal my body."

With my heart in my throat, I continued with bringing up the times where I hadn't spoken up for myself in relation to Ian. I was so far out of my comfort zone with admitting all of this. These admissions made me feel so vulnerable that the tears were flowing freely and my body was vibrating. After I had emptied out, there was silence. Then, it was Ian's turn. Ian also was not one to be confrontational, and it was just as uncomfortable for him to do this, but he did. Both our eyes were opened by this conversation, making me realize that life truly is all about perception. As it turned out, I had done or said things in the past that Ian perceived in a way that hurt him, which had not been my intent at all. Likewise, Ian had also said and done things to me in the past that I had misinterpreted.

About two hours later, when both of us had emptied out and cried and hugged, we felt lighter. Our relationship had just evolved a little and for that I was grateful.

45

Communication is really the crux of a great relationship and Ian and I made a commitment to each other right there in the car that we would keep this line of communication open from that point onward. Let's make our good relationship even better. However, the avoidance habit of covering my discomforts up with a smile proved to still be pretty powerful. Our commitment faltered more often than not, until our time in Malaysia.

I had discovered that the cancer was an indication that I was sitting on a proverbial minefield where numerous mines were hiding out, making it pretty dangerous territory. It was one of those "the more you know, the more you realize that you don't know" awarenesses. If I hadn't uncovered these mines, it would have been just a matter of time, in my opinion, before my body would have perished. My realization of the existence of this minefield was shortly after that fateful day in Malaysia when I received word that the cancer had spread.

By committing to my new surrendering practice, I made a pact with myself to delve into the unknown territory of this minefield. As I explored and surrendered at a conscious level, mines were being detonated, usually one at a time, but occasionally there were a couple that let go simultaneously. This exploration activated my emotional pain body, which had been dormant for so long. Although I was feeling pretty banged up while on this exploration mission, there were no lasting wounds, only relief, gratitude, compassion, and of course, love.

You can't surrender something if you're not even aware of its existence. This statement pretty much sums it up for me. When I was blissfully unaware, I was essentially blind to the fact that my programmed thoughts and beliefs were the root cause of the cancer, and therefore, not able to heal. Thankfully, I had some help pointing me in the right direction.

I remember how surprised I had been a year prior, when I first discovered in an Ayahuasca ceremony that I had low self-worth simply for being female. How could that be? I lived in a country where gender equality was pretty strong. I had an education. I had been a contributing provider in my family. Ian respected me. I was raised by a strong woman. I could go on and on. If I was struggling with that, I couldn't even imagine how other women around the world must feel. This was the first message that I received that indicated to me how oblivious I had been.

Did I really know who I even was at the core?

Another message that I received around the same time was that there would be a 100% chance of healing my body from cancer if I loved myself unconditionally. Love heals. My initial reaction to that one was, "But I do lots of things for myself. I exercise. I eat healthy. I do fun stuff. That's all loving myself, right?" Now I know that the undercurrent of those activities certainly were not based in love, not even close.

As I sit here, I realized that my surrendering journey took

me from blissfully unaware to painfully aware to ultimately becoming blissfully aware, over the span of about ten months. The bliss in blissfully unaware doesn't hold a candle to the bliss in blissfully aware, not even close. I will also admit that if I didn't have my motivational coach, aka cancer, in my corner throughout the painfully aware stage, I may very well have run for the hills. There were quite a few moments where I was not just taken, but thrown out of my comfort zone without a life vest. All I had was a trusting that this was the way to vibrant health. I endured despair, anger, fear, guilt, shame, and everything in between. It was no wonder I had become so skillful at avoiding shit, because it truly was shitty!

In the process of becoming blissfully aware, I discovered that the happiness that I had been feeling was a reaction to people, places, or experiences. In other words, that which was outside of myself and could come and go at the drop of a hat determined my level of happiness. I have found that there is much more depth in joy. Joy is a state of being that does not change just because the weather changes, someone doesn't want to be your friend anymore, or you lose your job. Joy is unconditional. Joy is the essence of being blissfully aware.

Cancer initially gifted me the strength to be relentless in my pursuit of making it with this beautiful body of mine. As time went on though, I felt that there was a strength within me that was blossoming. This inner strength is what I now tap into, and I know that it'll never let me down.

My suggestion to you would be to find your inner strength and do this for yourself, preferably before shit hits the fan in your life. Listen to the little nudges and go on your own exploration journey, just for the heck of it. You may just be surprised of what you'll find, like I was. And don't let the painfully aware stage stop you. Be strong, be committed, and be with it, because on the other side of the pain is eternal bliss. Eternal bliss! I promise you. It's there. Go for it! It will be the best thing you'll ever do for yourself and you are worthy of it.

PART 2

SURRENDERING TO VIBRANT HEALTH

In the following chapters I share with you my journey that took me from being blissfully unaware all the way to blissfully aware. It's my story of totally surrendering my emotional pain body through meditation.

A belief is just a thought that we keep on thinking. That doesn't make the belief true. It usually isn't.

Our reactions are triggered by our beliefs.

Pain is not caused by an event. It is caused by our reaction to an event. As a result, our beliefs can inadvertently create a lot of heartache and pain in our lives.

In other words, there are often heavy emotions and judgments that are attached to limiting beliefs. These heavy emotions and judgments are the resistance (reactions) that make the belief and coinciding events painful, putting our body in a state of dis-ease or stress.

Surrendering to the belief (being okay with it), releases the resistance to the incident or experience, which causes the pain to disappear, creating a state of ease in our body.

Thankfully, after doing lots of surrendering meditations on all the limiting beliefs that I had, I now feel a love for myself that is so gentle, so tender, and so compassionate that there are no words to describe its magnificence. And yes, there are still occasions where a limiting belief sneaks up, but I'm pretty quick to notice it and then surrender it. The more I do, the quicker I am able to surrender.

This is my story of how I became OKAY with all of my limiting beliefs, clearing the debris of heavy emotions which allowed me to then tune into my essence, LOVE.

Love healed my body, mind, and soul.

CHAPTER 7

The Power Of Belief

As I mentioned earlier, beliefs are just thoughts that we keep thinking. And so often, they're not true. In my case, I had many limiting, disempowering beliefs that I was unaware of until I started to put myself under the microscope. These beliefs programmed me to be a certain way. They were imbedded in me so deep that they actually festered and created tumours in my body. That's how powerful beliefs can be. Of course, I didn't set out in life wanting to believe these disempowering beliefs, but apparently, like most of us, I was a product of my environment.

The majority of these beliefs got their footing in my childhood. It helped me to know where these beliefs originated so that I could surrender at the deepest level. Surrendering these beliefs essentially deleted my programs so that I could start to reprogram myself in order to heal my body.

Anyone who has spent any time with me knows that I am incredibly bad with directions. I'm a pro at getting lost and have no confidence whatsoever in my directional sense. I decided to put the microscope on this, and asked myself a few questions.

How did I get to be so bad at directions? Why is it that I have no confidence whatsoever in myself when it comes to directions? Was I born this way or did something happen in my childhood that created this belief? What's interesting is that these questions took me to a memory of when I was about five years old where this belief and more may have been cemented into my cellular memory.

My family and I were visiting friends in a major Dutch city (I think it was The Hague) one day when all hell broke loose. My parents' friends had three sons. I had two brothers. All five of them were older and wanted nothing to do with me. I remember being bored and wanting to go to a nearby playground. My mother was busy helping with the dinner preparations and asked my father to take me. My father didn't really want to but took me anyway. He was never one to involve himself in playtime very much and this time was no different. He did not want to be there so he asked me if I knew how to get back to the house. I wanted him to stay but didn't feel comfortable asking him. I told him what he wanted to hear which was that I knew the way. He left me alone…at a playground in a major city. I was five years old.

Playing at the playground by myself wasn't much fun so I decided to go back, except I didn't remember which backyard gate to go through to get to our friends' house. They all looked the same to me. Being too shy to risk opening the wrong gate, I turned around and started walking out of the back alley and into the busy city. Thankfully two angels, in the forms of two little old ladies, stopped and asked me why I was crying and where my mommy was. They proceeded to take me to the police station. I had no idea what the family surname was of my parents' friends. All I knew was their first names and that they owned a clothing store. The police must have figured it out because after some time, my parents rushed in. My mother was crying and hugging me. I remember feeling very relieved, but also felt guilty for her tears and causing all this commotion. I don't remember how my father reacted. I avoided him out of fear that he'd be angry. Along with securing my belief of prone to getting lost, I'm pretty sure that my sense of rejection and abandonment started to take root as well on that day.

A few years later, another life changing belief cemented itself into my innocent subconscious. It was when my 37 year old mother was diagnosed with breast cancer. Back in the seventies, compared with present day, it was still quite uncommon for someone to be diagnosed with cancer at such a young age. I was about 8 years old at the time and didn't even really understand what cancer was, nor the seriousness of it, until I was biking home from school one day and was stopped by a man in the village who was asking me how my mother was doing. I told him that she was fine. He then felt the need to inform me, for whatever reason, that people usually die from cancer.

I was in shock and biked home in a daze. I was traumatized. Thankfully, my mother survived her first bout with cancer, but this experience had created a lot of fear within me. That, coupled with being told by many well-meaning people that I should get annual check-ups once I turned twenty, because there was a high chance that I'd get cancer too, cemented a belief system within the subconscious of my younger self that I was earmarked for this disease. In my opinion, this played a big role in the breast cancer diagnosis that I received at the age of 38, not because of genetics, but because of my belief system, along with mimicking my mother's behaviour.

I became aware of this notion a few years ago when I read the book The Biology of Belief by Dr. Bruce Lipton. It was the first time that I had heard of epigenetics and this concept empowered me like no other ever had. In his book, he explains that cells are primarily controlled by our beliefs. In other words, my beliefs have the ability to signal genes epigenetically and turn on or turn off the cancer cells in my body. This was a huge discovery in my world. Up until then, I believed, as did most people, that I was helpless when it came to cancer due to genetics. One doctor had even told me in 2007 that there was nothing I could have done differently in order to avoid it. He likely told me this so that I wouldn't blame myself. Instead, I felt so disempowered and victimized. I took that to mean that there was nothing I could do to prevent future diagnoses either, which put the fear of god into me. Dr. Bruce Lipton was a breath of fresh air for me. Thank you very much for making me feel empowered.

The next logical step was for me to access and change my subconscious belief system as well as uncover any mimicked self-limiting behaviours that I had taken on from my mother. Therein lay the problem. How on earth did I switch these babies off? Ayahuasca was good at bringing awareness to limiting beliefs and behaviours and definitely assisted in some of the letting go I did, but a lot of the inner subconscious work would have to be done in another way.

As I put myself under a microscope in all aspects of my life, I was somewhat surprised that I had definitely accumulated a fair amount of limiting beliefs that I hadn't been aware of before. Most of these disempowering beliefs caused me to play small instead of stepping out and seizing the moment. One of my favourite quotes is by Henry Ford. "Whether you think you can or you think you can't, you're right." It is such a powerful quote that, ironically, we had displayed on our wall at home for years. All those years I thought that my belief system was that of empowerment. How sneaky those subconscious beliefs could be!

It was humbling to say the least when I became aware of a subconscious disempowered belief that made me behave in a particular way that I had always despised. For years, I worked for the MS Society of Canada and spent quite a bit of time with my clients, several of whom were wheelchair bound. I enjoyed my job for the most part and truly saw my clients as friends. From time to time however, there was a type of behaviour that arose in some of them that annoyed me to no end.

I was well aware that my strong reaction to them meant that it was within myself as well. I called it victim energy. How I despise it! If I tried to empower certain clients a little too much, they would put me in my place. I'm sure that they didn't realize it, but it was as if their subconscious was saying to me, "Hang on. Don't empower me too much in that way. I've got power, thank you very much. It's called victim energy and it's pretty effective!" The idea that this resided within me as well made me squirm and filled with self-judgment. For the most part, I think I kept it under wraps except for one time (well, there were probably other times too, but this one stands out for me):

Our son was in grade twelve and preparations were made for his prom in the spring of 2017. Our small town did not have a facility big enough to hold over a hundred students and their family members for the dinner and dance that was organized every year by a group of volunteer parents. As a result, hundreds of combined parent volunteer hours were put in to transform an arena to a gorgeous venue fit for a prom. When our daughter graduated a couple of years earlier, both Ian and I took a week off work and contributed many, many hours. When our son graduated, however, I had already been diagnosed with cancer and was quite busy with my healing regime and getting better at saying no in order not to pile too much on my plate.

I only contributed one day of volunteering. The mother who I was assigned to volunteer with on the day that I helped was being quite nasty with me while I was volunteering. She didn't tell me why she was treating me so poorly, but I assumed that it was because she'd put in many hours and I hadn't done my share in her opinion. I allowed her to make me feel quite guilty and disempowered. At one point I said to her, "You know I have cancer, right?" Much to my chagrin, this question was filled with victim energy. She assured me that she did, continued to be rude with me, and eventually dismissed me.

I went to another area to help out where I felt significantly more appreciated. I was quite bothered that she could be so rude, but what really affected me about this incident was my choice to use the power of victim energy when I let her make me feel disempowered. Oh, did I beat myself up over that for weeks on end. That which I hated seeing in others had reared its ugly head in me. Ugh! This also had me wondering how many other times I used cancer to give me the power of victim energy at a subconscious level. After all, cancer got me much craved attention. I didn't have to go to work because of the diagnosis. People did things for me that they otherwise may not have, etc. Then, I looked at this through the eyes of my father's daughter and bingo! I got to the root of it.

As I mentioned earlier, my mother was diagnosed with cancer twice in her lifetime. Both times, my father was very supportive, but his caregiver role increased exponentially with my mother's second diagnosis when they were told that her cancer was terminal. My father loved her dearly and there was nothing he wouldn't do for her as a caregiver. They sold the farm and he retired for the time being so that he could focus all of his attention on her. His attention was something that I was not privy to and craved more than I ever realized.

Subconsciously I must have thought that a cancer diagnosis would result in that kind of attention from him. Alas, that did not happen, and he continued to reject me. In the search for attention elsewhere, along with other behaviour strategies, I played the victim card at times. Sometimes it was subtle while other times it was probably glaringly obvious. Either way, I was usually somewhat aware of it and there was no shortage of judgments that I had for myself in this regard.

Our belief systems can make or break us. I was hovering around the breaking point, definitely too close for comfort. Thankfully, I caught myself at the eleventh hour and got catapulted into the zone where magic of epic proportions is possible.

The Journey provided the tools I needed to get to the cellular memory of my traumatic experiences. I had numerous Journey sessions that uncovered and released several of the limiting beliefs I had. I'm grateful for what they did for me. There were some challenges however. The only way to do a Journey session is with a partner. On top of that, I was in really bad shape and knew that I had a lot of shit to let go of. Time and money played a factor. And finally, I was traveling around Asia and didn't always have great wifi.

Thankfully, I came up with a solution. I call it the Surrendering Meditation. This meditation gave me back my life and so much more!

Interested in doing a Surrendering Meditation?

Find a quiet place where there'll be no distractions.

Sit or lie down comfortably. Close your eyes. Music is optional.

Bring up the limiting belief you want to surrender and truly feel all the heavy emotions that are attached to this belief. You can intensify it even more by bringing up certain memories related to this limiting belief or thinking of the worst case scenario (you may start to cry, shiver, sweat, or none of the above. Let it all happen without judgments).

Once you feel it fully, hold space for it by saying,

"It's OK." repeatedly. Be patient and let go of any expectations for the emotions to dissipate. Ironically, letting go of expectations is exactly what's required for the emotions to dissipate.

When you feel yourself lighten up, gratitude, love, compassion, and forgiveness may arise within you. This could take 5 minutes, 30 minutes, or longer.

Bathe yourself in all of these high vibrational feelings for as long as possible.

Your body is now in a state of ease. This is the sweet spot where lots of healing happens.

This is where you know that you are invincible!

Now take a moment to visualize the incident the way that you'd like for it to be, feeling as if it has already happened.

If you're wondering if you've fully surrendered the limiting belief, you can test it out by putting yourself in a position where you're experiencing an event that used to trigger a reaction out of you. If there's no reaction, great!

If you still feel a bit triggered, meditate on it again.

Repeat until it has completely neutralized.

"It's OK" are the words spoken by your higher consciousness. It's beckoning your ego to let go of your resistance to the heavy emotions.

This neutralizes the emotions attached to the limiting belief, dissipating the belief, making the event or experience a non-issue.

When it's a non-issue, we are no longer stressing about it. Instead, we are in a state of ease.

The more at ease that we are, the more we are able to feel our true essence, LOVE.

If you feel somewhat doubtful about this process, think about a time that you had a good cry. Feeling better after a good cry is something that most of us are familiar with. This is really no different. The only difference is that it's done with intention and with added ammunition of really super charging the emotions.

It's important that no one tries to calm you down or give you a hug while you're in the throes of it. Even when that is done with the best intention, it can really alter the momentum and the intensity level of the healing. It needs to run its course without interference in order for optimum results. Be sure to ask your loved ones to surrender their need to interfere.

CHAPTER 8

Falling Apart In Paradise

The surrendering process sometimes came in stages for me. For example, I'd feel something come up during meditation and surrender to it, then later that day, I would get triggered in one way or another and it was time to take it to the next level. I would stop whatever I was doing and let it all pour out. And yes, the timing was usually crappy, but I knew that it was best to surrender in that moment while it was fresh.

In October of 2018, I was hanging out in gorgeous tropical Malaysia where, as I mentioned before, my inner world had crumbled overnight upon receiving the message of apparent doom (aka stage 4 cancer). I felt like a zombie, just going through the motions. I was surrounded by such stunning nature, and yet, I was in such a state of inner turmoil that I may as well have been in a dark cave.

But like I said before, I was committed. There would be no backing down, no stuffing down emotions. The avoidance game had to be a thing of the past. Not only had I set the intention to surrender to everything that came to the surface, I was also super aware of every little thought, feeling, or emotion that passed through my mind. Nothing got by me. I was like a hawk. Bring it on!

Body...show me what you've got!

I got shown alright! First up, anger. I didn't do anger very well at all. Anger had definitely not been in my repertoire. Still, there it was, bubbling up inside of me. It was a tough one for me. We didn't do anger at home and considering that society kind of frowns upon it as well, I tended to avoid it at all cost. However, I continually reminded myself of the promise I had made to myself to sit with whatever came up to the surface. So come hell or high water, I was doing it.

The anger that came up initially (yes, initially, meaning that it was a pretty common emotion that I had to surrender to over and over again at different levels) was about the unfairness of it all. Being in the prime of my life and yet, bending over backwards to stay alive...really? Had I been a heavy smoker, drinker, sedentary junk food eater kind of person, I probably would have been a little more accepting of my situation, but the fact that I was none of those things made it a pretty tough pill to swallow. It was a pill that I had previously not allowed myself to acknowledge. The time had come. It was time to acknowledge and surrender this anger.

How? Meditation.

I sat comfortably with my eyes closed and soft music playing into my head phones.

I set my intention: surrender the unfairness of having cancer.

I brought up all the emotions that were attached to this belief that it was unfair. I didn't hold back; I felt it thoroughly. I magnified it. Thoughts like "Life is unfair! I have a right to be angry! I hate cancer! It sucks to be sick!" surfaced. These thoughts brought the results that I was looking for - it intensified the anger. I wanted it to consume me, to overwhelm me. My body temperature was rising. I was shaking like a leaf. I was crying. In other words, I was a mess and, believe it or not, that's exactly what I wanted. I knew that my body was releasing all the pent up anger, and even as intense as it was, I persevered.

Then, I told myself over and over again, "IT'S OK that I feel anger. IT'S OK that I feel anger. IT'S OK that I feel anger. IT'S OK. IT'S OK. IT'S OK!" I said this over and over again. Finally, it burned itself out and left my body. Crying, sweating, and shaking are the body's ways of releasing emotions. Surrendering to all of that was vital. When I eventually stopped crying, shaking, and sweating, I knew that the anger was lifted out of me, into the light of love. I knew when it was gone because I started to feel more relaxed in my body. I could breathe easier, the knot in my stomach had disappeared, and my throat no longer felt constricted. I felt a loving, compassionate gentleness wash over me that I hadn't felt before. I bathed in this loving energy for as long as possible, knowing that this loving energy had the power to heal me while feeling lots of gratitude for it.

In other words, when I became 100% okay with my anger, my belief that it was unfair for me to have cancer at such a young age became a nonissue and I was okay with it. I realized that I had in fact not ever allowed myself to fully feel anger, always stuffing it down and that was the real issue. This surrendering meditation allowed me to finally embrace this anger with love. It allowed me to embody love.

I'm guessing that you're probably not going to be too surprised about the next biggie that needed to be surrendered. Fear of dying. Again, this was something that I had avoided. (Notice a pattern here?) When this doozy came up, I actually realized that it wasn't fear of dying, but fear of pain while dying that I needed to surrender.

My mother had endured a very painful death that lasted several years. She died from stage 4 breast cancer that had spread to her bones. This type of cancer causes the bones to become very weak and break easily. Small bones break the easiest, such as the ribs (that can't be casted) and cause a lot of pain when broken. Something as seemingly innocent as a sneeze or a cough could snap a bone. My family and I felt desperately helpless as we watched my mom being eaten up by cancer, and it left its mark on all of us. No, I wasn't afraid of death. After all, I knew with utmost certainty that we do not die; we just continue on in a different realm. However, I had an incredible fear of pain while dying, because I had witnessed my mother go through it.

As I mentioned before, this one was a doozy to surrender. Embracing the emotion of fear was one thing, but embracing the notion of pain was quite another. However, I knew that the importance of surrendering this was two-fold. One, releasing this fear obviously was good at an emotional level; and two, surrendering to pain would also allow my body to let go of tension. Seeing that tension tends to increase the pain, this was an important aspect to consider. It may have been a tough one, but I was determined to let this fear go.

In the throes of surrendering to the fear of pain, I once again was crying and shaking, but instead of sweating, I was shivering. This is another way that the body releases blocked energy. Something else that was happening for me was I had a constant need to yawn. Yawning also releases energy.

This surrendering meditation took significantly longer. I would start to relax a little, thinking that the worst had passed, only for the fear to surge back and overwhelm me even more. This had a lot of cellular memory attached to it, making me realize that a Journey process would be very beneficial in helping me surrender to it.

In the Journey process I was taken back by way of a guided meditation to the time of the event when I developed the intense fear of pain. It was when I watched my mother suffer from horrendous pain while dying from cancer. With the help of a practitioner who guided me in this somewhat structured process, I released the cellular memory that was attached to the fear. Of course, no one wants to experience pain, and I was no exception. But, after the Journey process, the fear didn't quite have the stronghold on me anymore. In other words, it no longer consumed me. I was getting free.

This was just the beginning of my surrendering practice while in paradise. I continued down this path for the duration of my time in Asia and beyond. As a matter of fact, my surrendering practice is a life time commitment. Thankfully, it does get easier with time.

Chapter 9

My Father: One Of My Greatest Masters

As children, we're like sponges. We take everything at face value and believe it to be true. Whatever people say to us or how they treat us has the power to create lifelong beliefs of ourselves and how we perceive the world. The people who raise us, most often our parents, usually have the biggest impact. Therefore, if we are bullied or made to feel disempowered in our childhood, having nothing to weigh up against it, no previous experience to counter it, we are likely to believe that we, in fact, have no power. These beliefs often stay with us and become the cornerstone for our thoughts and behaviour throughout our lives and eventually these beliefs mould into our personality.

Keeping this in mind, through the help of meditation, Journey work, and plant medicine, I discovered the root causes of my behaviours and thought patterns that were tucked away in my subconscious. They were subtle enough that I was completely oblivious to them for most of my life. I was oblivious because I didn't know any better. After all, I'd been that way for decades so it was my *normal*. I believed "this is just the way I am."

This programming, and that's exactly what it is, can be altered. We all have the ability to reprogram ourselves, but as I found out, it takes persistence and the will for change. This is not for the faint of heart. Reprogramming yourself essentially means that you are recreating yourself and your life, causing you to step out of your norm, aka your comfort zone, and step into the river of the unknown. You will probably feel all kinds of resistance and the people around you are likely to put up a bit of a stink too, because you no longer will be who they expect you to be. But if you persevere, the payoff can be amazing. That's what happened to me.

But first, I need to set the foundation. Seeing that I was raised by my parents, they had the biggest impact on my life. There was my mother, who was gentle and loving, and then there was my father, a strong man who had a heart of gold, but...

My father has been one of the greatest masters in my life. I would not be where I am today if it wasn't for him and for that I am eternally grateful. Along with cancer, my father is the biggest reason of why I finally made the life saving decision to dig deep and find my inner strength. In other words, what he did was for me, not to me.

My father was a bully. Like most bullies, he was initially a shy boy who was bullied himself by the kids at school. Bullied, until one fateful day, when on the advice of his father, he made the choice to stand up for himself on the playgrounds of his elementary school. Up until then, he hadn't realized his physical strength. When he discovered the power of his punch, he went to every kid that had ever bullied him in the past and beat them in a fist fight. Apparently, there had been quite a few kids on this list, considering that my father was eventually expelled from the school playground. He was to arrive only when the school bell rang and was not allowed to linger after school. This event marked a pivotal time in my father's life that was to set the tone in most of his future relationships.

I can imagine the amazing feeling of power that he must have felt as a ten year old boy, finally beating those kids who had bullied him and made him feel disempowered for years. I can fully understand how he would never want to put himself in that position of vulnerability again. In the end, he had shown those kids who was boss and with that, he had successfully stopped all bullying attempts towards him. Unfortunately, this survival mechanism did not differentiate between would-be bullies and the rest of society. As a result, the minute my father felt even a little bit threatened by anyone, he would attack.

Although he eventually outgrew his fist fights, he became

more savvy with his bullying methods in his adult years. From my perspective, he was intense and used intimidation to overpower others. I have often said that he should have been a lawyer. Very few could stand up to him, including myself. Someone recently gave me the analogy of some people only having a hammer in their toolbox. This was definitely true with regard to my father.

I do want to point out that when my father was not feeling threatened, and when things were going his way, he was a loving father. He was also a great provider who took his role as a father and husband seriously. He provided a roof over our heads and made sure that we didn't go without. Throughout our childhood, my brothers and I played sports, took music lessons, hung out with our friends, and went on annual family vacations. My father could be the life of the party and a lot of fun to be around. There is no doubt in my mind that my father loved us, albeit conditionally. Our life at home was pretty ideal...as long as no one rocked the boat.

I was a feisty toddler and with the need to show me who was boss, my father overpowered me from the get-go. He bullied me into submission and turned me into a people pleaser. I became an expert at not rocking the boat. As you may expect, I wasn't the only one in my family who perfected this survival skill. It was rare that any of us stood up and challenged my father, least of all myself. When I finally did, however, it would turn into an event of epic proportions that lasted ten years.

It was Christmas of 2003 and our first Christmas without my mom, who had passed away from cancer earlier that year. That alone made it a heart wrenching time. Add to that the beginning of the end of my 'people pleasing, don't rock the boat' relationship with my father, and I was an emotional wreck.

It started with the crumbling of an already unstable relationship between my husband, Ian, and my father. I had felt the tension between them for years, and it became apparent that my mother had been the glue that held it together. At the beginning of their deteriorating relationship, I was caught in the middle, feeling incredibly anxious. The one thing that I avoided like the plague, the one thing that I couldn't handle, was happening...turmoil in my precious little world where those I loved were unable to get along with each other. Try as I might, I was unable to fix that which ended up being unfixable. After a few very stressful and awkward months where my father was filled with judgments, I wrote an email to him and finally stood up for myself and Ian. I risked rocking the boat. It took a lot out of me to find the courage to send this email but with my heart in my throat, I hit 'send'.

As fate would have it, my father felt under attack and the bully showed up in spades. His reply was incredibly hurtful and shocked me to the core. The people pleaser in me was devastated. I sent him another email, begging for him to see my perspective and to agree to disagree with me, but he would have none of it. He continued to be harsh and hurtful. As a result, much to my horror, we did not bury the hatchet for almost ten years, but not for lack of trying on my part. How could my own father just write me off like that? I was devastated.

In 2018, I did a surrendering meditation to heal my relationship with my father.

I sat comfortably with my eyes closed and soft music playing into my head phones.

I set my intention: surrender my relationship with my father.

I brought up all the emotions that were attached to rejection. I didn't hold back. I felt it thoroughly. I magnified it. I allowed myself to cry. I allowed myself to be angry. I allowed myself to feel hurt. I felt it all with gusto.

Then, I told myself over and over again, "IT'S OK that I feel this fear of rejection. IT'S OK that I feel this fear of rejection. IT'S OK that I feel this fear of rejection. IT'S OK. IT'S OK. IT'S OK." I said this over and over again until the fear was lifted out of me into the light of love. I knew when it was gone because I started to feel more relaxed in my body. I could breathe easier. The knot in my stomach had disappeared, and I no longer had a lump in my throat. I felt a loving, compassionate gentleness wash over me that I hadn't felt before. I bathed in this loving energy for as long as possible, knowing that this loving energy had the power to heal me.

Fear of rejection was deeply entrenched within me and required numerous surrendering meditations for all the layers to dissipate.

When I became 100% okay with my fear of rejection, rejection by my father became a nonissue and I was okay with it. I realized that I had, in fact, rejected myself all these years and this was the real issue allowing me to finally embrace myself unconditionally.

CHAPTER 10

My First Cancer Diagnosis

May 2007 marked the first time that I received the devastating news. I had been having routine mammograms for years and this year was no different. We usually combined these appointments in the city with other activities and often made a weekend out of it. With Ian and the kids waiting in the car, I went in for my check-up that year with the assumption that it would just be a quick in-and-out appointment. Not this time. The mammogram was showing something that they wanted to have a closer look at, so an ultrasound was next on the docket. The ultrasound technician then called for a radiologist to have a look.

At this point, I had started to freak out a little on the inside. When the radiologist suggested that he wanted me to come back after lunch so that he could perform a biopsy,

I may have stopped breathing. The fear that crept up in me was shaking me to the core. I put my clothes back on and numbly walked out into the waiting room.

Ian had parked the car and come inside, wondering what was taking me so long. The lump in my throat was so thick that I couldn't speak. I didn't have to; it was written all over my face. Ian wrapped his arms around me and we stood there, in the waiting room, numb with shock. Could it be? Needing to pull ourselves together for our kids, I took some deep breaths and fiercely pushed down the fears.

The ten days that followed were some of the longest days ever. Not knowing is almost worse than knowing the results. I numbly went through the motions, walking around in a daze, but telling no one about my fears.

A tumour was indeed found in my left breast. At the age of 38, I heard the dreaded words that no one wants to hear. "You have cancer."

Life was pretty much a blur after that. I was scheduled for a bunch more tests, including a bone scan to rule out any other hot spots. I met with the surgeon and had a lumpectomy within a couple of weeks. I was told that it was stage 1 so it was unlikely that I would need chemotherapy. The surgery was successful, but it came with some unfortunate news. They had discovered that there was vascular invasion meaning that cancer cells were found on the walls of my veins. This also meant that there was a high risk of those cancer cells breaking away from the vein walls and flowing freely through my body. In other words, there could be cancer in my big toe for all they knew, and chemotherapy would ensure that any of those potential floaties would be poisoned to death.

I had come to terms with surgery and radiation, but chemotherapy was a whole other ballgame in my opinion. The oncologist gave me a week to decide whether I would choose chemo or not. That week was nerve wracking as I agonized over the decision. I flip-flopped back and forth, depending on the day, who I'd talked to, and what my frame of mind was. Ian assured me that he would support me in whatever decision I chose. It was up to me. If it had been just about me, I would not have chosen chemotherapy. That's how much I was against it. The thought of there being possible cancer cells floating around my vascular system made me realize, however, that I didn't want to risk the possibility of leaving Ian as a single dad while our young kids grew up without a mom. By the end of the week, I reached a decision. I chose chemotherapy, not for me but for them.

After almost three years of not communicating with my father, I wrote him a letter, letting him know of my diagnosis. Considering the experience he had through supporting my mom while she battled cancer, I told him that I needed him in my life. Once again, I asked him if we could agree to disagree and let bygones be bygones. His reply came in the mail on the very day that I had my first chemo treatment. Feeling nauseous and weak from the treatment, I sat outside in our back yard and read his letter. By the time I finished reading the letter, I was weeping uncontrollably. He had rejected me, yet again, and I was devastated. Ian stepped in, angrily took the letter out of my hands and ripped it into a thousand pieces before throwing it in the garbage. "We are done with your father!" he exclaimed. "We have enough on our plate without him!" I agreed and vowed that I would never reach out to him again, that I was in fact done with him forever as well.

Little did I know then that I would never be able to get over him. But, there would come a time, about six years down the road where there would be a deep healing within me, which would not have happened if my father had accepted my numerous pleas of reconciliation earlier.

This deep inner healing happened at my first Ayahuasca retreat in Mexico in November of 2013. How did Ayahuasca cross the path of someone like me…a farm girl who had never really been into drugs and had not even heard of this thing called Ayahuasca? Well, for that, I need to backtrack to January of that year, when I came across the book entitled When The Body Says No: The Link Between Stress And Chronic Illness by Dr. Gabor Maté. This book turned out to be pivotal in my life. I had a-ha moment after a-ha moment and saw myself and my mother in many of the palliative care patients that Dr. Maté had interviewed for his book. To top it all off, there was a repressed memory that came to the surface while I was reading the book.

I'm not sure what triggered this memory, but there it was. It shook me to the core. "How had I not remembered this?" I thought to myself. It was a memory of sexual inappropriateness from my childhood, a term that Gabor later disagreed with. He told me that it wasn't just inappropriate; it was abuse. Either way, I was about twelve years old and my breasts were starting to develop. There was an adult who was very interested in this development and asked to see them and measure them on a regular basis. This unwanted attention made me very uncomfortable and self conscious. I guess it would now be called sexual harassment. In any case, the fact that I was just an innocent child, awkward enough as it was in my developing body, it did enough damage that I blocked that memory for more than thirty years. Thankfully, after we moved to Canada, this harassment stopped, but the damage was done. I hated my body, including my breasts, for decades to come.

This memory and the a-ha moments were enough for me to know that I needed to meet this Dr. Gabor Maté. Despite my supervisor's assurance that my performance at work was great, I had already decided prior to reading this book that I wasn't busy enough at work, and wanted to create an additional fundraising event. As fate would have it, Dr. Gabor Maté was also a keynote speaker and was available to come to my small home town that spring to do a presentation called "When The Body Says No".

Not only was this event a huge success as well as a great fundraiser, it was literally the best thing I could have done for my own evolvement as well. I had the pleasure of taking Gabor out for dinner prior to the event where our topic of conversation inevitably went to the effects of stress on our health. He asked me how I was, to which I replied with a big smile that I was doing great. I was more interested in asking him for advice in regard to my daughter's hair pulling.

"When did she start that?" he asked.

"When I was diagnosed with cancer six years ago" was my reply.

"And you say that you're fine?" was his response.

My smile faltered a little as I started to feel a little uncomfortable. "Well...I could relate a lot to what you wrote in your book," I said. And upon giving him a quick Coles notes version of my life history, Gabor told me that he ran a retreat in Mexico where Ayahuasca was used to help people with their healing journey. He proceeded to tell me that I was a prime candidate, and that if I was interested, he would put in a good word for me to be accepted, as they often sold out. Having never heard of Ayahuasca, my curiosity was piqued. When the dust settled post-event, I turned to Google and started my research.

My immediate reaction was "What!? A psychedelic drug? Holy cow! I don't do drugs." This was so beyond anything I had ever done that it freaked me out. Ian, on the other hand, didn't seem phased at all and calmly asked me if I trusted Dr. Maté. I didn't have to ponder that question long at all, "Yes, I definitely feel that I can trust him."

"Then you should go", Ian replied. "It's time that you deal with your fear of cancer and your relationship with your dad."

"But we can't afford for me to go!" I replied, to which Ian quietly responded in a way that I'll never forget.

"We can't afford for you not to go".

Wow, that got my attention! Apparently I had not fooled Ian either, for he knew that under my smiley facade, there was a roller coaster of emotions that hovered around fear and lack of self worth. Apparently, the time had come for me to start the inner work.

Ian's comment sealed the deal. I contacted Gabor and filled out my application for my first retreat with Ayahuasca. Little did I know then the impact Ayahuasca would have on my life. I am forever grateful that Dr. Gabor Maté came into my life when he did. His guidance alongside Ayahuasca turned out to be pivotal.

The retreat consisted of three Ayahuasca ceremonies tucked into a week of meditations, journaling, eating a special diet, and of course, daily group sessions with Gabor. I remember being quite nervous in preparation of the first ceremony, but felt safe in the hands of a great shaman and his helpers. Nothing could have prepared me for the experience that I was about to have, for it was so beyond my scope. During that ceremony, there were moments where I let go of grief that I didn't even know was still stored in my body. Ayahuasca also showed me that I was not my mother and that her fate with cancer did not pre-determine my fate with cancer.

It was also in this ceremony that I was able to change my perspective of my father. For the first time, I saw how my father was a product of his environment. He had been born in war-torn Europe in 1939 where fear and anger were the ruling vibrations throughout the world. Along with that, his father was incapable of loving and was quite abusive. Then, there was the bullying at school. Was it any wonder that my father's survival technique was that of aggression? For the first time I was able to let go of all the judgments, anger, and hurt that I had felt towards him for all these years. Instead, I felt compassion for my father. I knew that it wasn't about forgiveness, for who was I to need him to be anything other than who he was? He was on his own journey and after all, at some level I chose him to be a part of my journey. Along with compassion, feelings of love and gratitude now arose within me.

I remember telling Gabor that I was going to write my father a letter to let him know that I still loved him and wanted to reconnect with him. "You know that your father may still reject you?" he said. "He wasn't here at this retreat; he didn't do the inner work."

"Yes", I agreed, "he likely will reject me again, and that's okay. I now know that if he does, it's because of fear, and I won't take it personally." Needless to say I was more than surprised when I received a response from my father about a month later where he agreed to reconnect with me.

It had been ten whole years and we finally had a chance to patch things up. It started with emails. Then, we agreed to talk on the phone. My father, who was known to overpower, let me talk my heart out. That first phone conversation was deep and a lot of healing happened. I wasn't looking for an apology. I remembered my mother telling me years ago to not ever expect an apology from my father. At that time, I didn't understand it. "Don't we all make mistakes, and wouldn't we all want to make it better by apologizing?" I've since come to the realization that bullies will do anything in their power to avoid feeling vulnerable. Apologizing is a pretty big act of vulnerability. Most bullies wouldn't touch that with a ten foot pole!

After a few more phone conversations, I felt that I was ready to fly out and visit with my father in Eastern Canada. Both our kids wanted to come along, too, so that they could spend time with their cousins. Having no desire to rekindle his relationship with my father, Ian did not come along. My father had no interest in reconnecting with Ian either, and I was at peace with that. At least they agreed on one thing!

Leading up to the visit, I was feeling nervous and anxious. The visit went better than expected though. The dynamics of our relationship had definitely taken a turn for the better. Not once did my father try to bully me. How could that be? And, how was it that my father had shut me down twice when I had reached out in the past, but when I had done the inner work this time around, he welcomed me back into his life? Coincidence? I think not. It would be years before I realized the real answers to those questions.

I eventually learned that we are all connected at an energetic level. Imagine that this energetic connection is a cord that, in this case, spans between my father and I. By feeling compassion, love, and gratitude for my father instead of anger, hurt, and judgments, I had cleared up my end of this energetic cord and heightened the vibration. My father may not have been conscious of this cleaned up vibration, but I'm sure that he felt it at a subconscious level, which lowered his defences and prompted him to agree to reconnect with me. Gabor was right about one thing. My father had not been at the retreat on a physical level, but energetically, he had been there in spades!

Chapter 11

Fear Of Rejection

My father and I were on speaking terms again. Problem fixed, right? Oh, if only it could have been that easy. Unfortunately, this ten year hiatus between us added fuel to an already strong feeling of rejection that had been present within me since childhood.

This feeling of rejection took root decades earlier, when, at the tender age of thirteen, I immigrated with my family in 1982 to Canada from the Netherlands. Although initially excited about the adventure of moving to a different continent, reality hit pretty hard when we landed in this beautiful, vast country where they spoke a language that was all but foreign to me. I was already quite awkward to begin with, but being plunked into a grade seven classroom without a life vest proved to be terrifying. It did not take me very long to learn English; that wasn't the problem. The other students definitely made an attempt at getting to know me at first, so that wasn't the problem either. There were some wonderful teachers at this school who went out of their way to help me in this transition, eliminating that as a problem as well. What was the problem then?

I didn't fit in.

Plain and simple. I was miserable and would have crawled back to the Netherlands on my hands and knees if they'd let me. I was homesick for more than two years. Although I was never diagnosed at that time, I now know that I was struggling with depression. I was lonely, and I felt isolated. I was too proud to tell my parents, nor did I want to rock the boat, so I suffered in silence. I remember lying in bed at night, crying and wishing for me to be more outgoing at school. "All I want is to be Jennie's friend" was one of many silent pleas that went through my head during those days.

The truth was, I had crawled into a shell and didn't know how to come out. I was very self-conscious and awkward. I barely spoke to anyone at school. Thankfully, after about a year, I did meet Shelley, a very outgoing, wonderful girl from a different school who took me under her wing and played a big role in making my life more bearable outside of school.

When I graduated from the Florenceville Intermediate

School in 1984, and got ready to start high school, I made a pact with myself to make friends. A new school, new students, and a new and improved me, I was determined to crawl out of this shell and find a way to fit in and be liked. And I did. I blossomed. Not only did I make new friends, but I also started dating and had my first boyfriend. Life was good again and I was able to put the past behind me, for the time being.

It's funny how the past can creep back to haunt us in ways that we never expect. The school wallflower experience had left a mark within me that I only just became aware of not so long ago. While at a Journey retreat in the Netherlands during the summer of 2018, I learned about the Enneagram, a system that teaches nine different personality types and how they can affect emotions and behaviour. I registered as a 7.

What does this have to do with anything?

Our childhood experiences program us to behave a certain way. I was painfully shy and felt invisible as a young teenager. I hated being that way, and did whatever I could to be the total opposite. I became a type 7 on the Enneagram chart. In other words, the wallflower experience had ignited fear in me. Fear of not being heard. Fear of not being seen. Fear of not being liked.

I reacted to this fear by overcompensating. This is part of the personality type 7. When those feelings of rejection, being unloved, invisible, and unheard were brought back up to the surface when my relationship with my father fell apart, I started behaving in ways that brought attention to me. Again, this was all done at a subconscious level. I was oblivious for the most part that I was doing this, and had no idea that the root cause of this behaviour was fear.

Some of the behaviours I exhibited were that I started to overpower conversations and talk people's ears off, out of fear that I would otherwise go unheard. I also started wearing more vibrant and form-fitting clothing with lots of jewelry, out of fear that I would otherwise become invisible again. My people pleasing efforts skyrocketed out of fear that I would not be loved otherwise. And last but not least, I started looking for love in all the wrong places.

My tendency to talk too much was something I had been aware of for some time and I used to beat myself up over it. A couple of my more introverted friends were okay with it. They would tell me how much they appreciated me at a party for keeping the conversation going so that they didn't have to worry about giving too much input. However, I was also told the opposite and that some people thought that my personality was over the top and annoying. To be honest, there were times when I would meet someone who could out-talk me, and I would realize how annoying and exhausting that could be as a bystander. When I recognized myself in these people, I didn't like it one little bit.

In my early thirties, around the time that my relationship

with my father deteriorated, I started putting more effort into my appearance. I grew my hair a bit to look more feminine and started wearing more vibrant and form fitting clothes. I was often told by other women how much they liked my style of clothing, which of course fed my ego. In and of itself, changing one's style is pretty harmless, but once again, the undercurrent of my behaviour was that of fear. I was afraid that I would otherwise not be noticed.

Neither of these behaviours are earth shattering, however, when combined with everything else that I did, it added another drop to the bucket of my unhealthy inner world. It was worth paying attention to and adding it to my ever-growing surrendering list.

Here is the meditation I did in 2018 to deal with this issue.

I sat comfortably with my eyes closed and soft music playing into my head phones.

I set my intention: surrender my need to be seen and heard.

I brought up all the emotions that were attached to this fear of not being seen or heard. I didn't hold back. I took myself back to when I was that wallflower. I felt the fear thoroughly. I magnified it. I allowed myself to cry. I allowed myself to feel shame. I allowed myself to feel guilt. I felt it all with gusto!

Then, I told myself over and over again, "IT'S OK that I feel this fear of being invisible and unheard. IT'S OK that I feel this fear of being invisible and unheard. IT'S OK that I feel this fear of being invisible and unheard. IT'S OK. IT'S OK. IT'S OK." I said this over and over again until the fear was lifted out of me into the light of love. I knew when it was gone because I started to feel more relaxed in my body. I could breathe easier, and the knot in my stomach had disappeared. I no longer had a lump in my throat. I felt a loving, compassionate gentleness wash over me that I hadn't felt earlier. I bathed in this loving compassionate energy for as long as possible, knowing that this loving energy had the power to heal me.

In other words, when I became 100% okay with my fear of being invisible and unheard, it became a nonissue and I was okay with it. I realized that I had, in fact, made myself small and insignificant all these years and that this was the real issue. This surrendering meditation allowed me to finally see, hear, and love myself.

When arriving back in Canada after spending more than eight months in hot and humid Asia, I went shopping for warmer clothes. After coming home with my purchases, I noticed that I had bought a grey jean jacket, grey pants, grey shoes, and a black sports jacket. Hmmm, interesting. I usually made a point of not wearing those colours, because they were too blah in my opinion. Then, I made the connection. Oh yeah! I had let go of the fear of not being seen.

Will I only be wearing grey and black clothing from now on? Absolutely not! I still love the beautiful, vibrant colours of the colour wheel, but I now wear them with the energy of self love instead of needing to be seen.

CHAPTER 12

Our Unconventional Marriage

Ian and I started dating during the summer of 1988 while we were both working at a resort in Western Canada. I was still a student at Acadia University in Eastern Canada and had three years left before graduation. There was about 5000 kilometres between us, making it a pretty long distance relationship while I was at school. We decided to give it a try with the option to date other people while apart, and being monogamous during the summers while we were together. We figured that if our relationship was meant to be then it would work out.

We married in 1995, and kept it monogamous for approximately ten years before choosing to make it an open relationship again. This happened around the same time that my relationship with my father fell apart. I had not ever looked at the timing of this until now. Could that be a coincidence? Probably not.

It was initially Ian's suggestion to open up our marriage and give it a try. After all, it had worked all those years before. It took a bit of convincing, but I eventually came on board with it, and even enjoyed it. Ian and I have never felt jealousy for each other in our relationship so we knew that we didn't have to worry about that aspect. The premise of our open relationship was that we loved each other unconditionally and that we had enough love in us to expand our horizons, so to speak.

We lived in a small town. Ian was an elected public official and one of my jobs was that of a teacher. Along with that, we had two children. You can imagine that it was important to us that we keep this a secret in order to avoid a scandal. Thankfully, we were able to successfully keep it under wraps, until now of course. We had busy lives with work and kids so the opportunities of get togethers with others were minimal. However, as time went on, I became more and more adventurous and promiscuous. No, it's not that I was with a different man every weekend, not even close. However, there were a few.

Most of the time, these men were kind and respectful towards me. Much like a normal date, we would meet for dinner and get to know each other first. In the beginning it was exciting and I thrived on all the attention that I received from these men. This was attention that I was craving in order to make me feel whole and lovable. But, in one incident, the people pleaser in me got me in a hot mess.

I'd known for a while that I was a people pleaser and that it didn't always serve me well. Not being able to say no is a pretty common trait of a people pleaser, and I was one with a capital P. I remember hanging out with a dear friend of mine at an event several years before when a lady came over to ask my friend if she would be willing to volunteer for something at her kids' school. My friend's reply was simply "no". She did not say sorry. She did not give an explanation. She just said "no". The woman did not seem offended. She said, "OK", and wandered off.

I was amazed! Just say no? You can do that? Without telling her why? Wow! I needed to take some notes! How many times had I agreed to do something that I would have rather not done simply because I couldn't say "no"?

It's been said that we rarely make a change until we've hit rock bottom, when the only way to go is up. This next experience took me over the edge, so to speak.

...Okay, I'm procrastinating...I need to take a big breath here before I continue. You see, this is probably where I've had to dig the deepest within myself to get to a place where I'm okay with sharing this experience with you. There was so much shame with this one that I've had to work through. You see, I wasn't young and foolish at the time that this happened. No, I was a middle-aged woman, a wife, a mother of two, yada yada yada. A woman who seemingly had herself pulled together in such a way that you'd assume she would have learned the skills of standing up for herself and definitely would have learned to say, "No!"

I met with a man who ended up being much older than he had told me. I should have clued into that when we Face Timed prior to our rendezvous. He sat in the sun at such an angle that I could only see his silhouette. As I walked into the restaurant on the night of this rendezvous, to meet him for dinner, I remember standing by the entrance as he walked towards me. My thoughts were somewhere along the lines of "Holy cow, that's him?"

He was definitely not in his fifties, probably not even in his sixties. He lied about his age. "He is too old for me. Get me out of here." was all I could think. My mind was going a mile a minute, however being the person that I was, I didn't let on that I was upset at all and put on my smiley mask.

We had made the agreement ahead of time that if I wasn't feeling the vibe, that I could back out, no questions asked, and of course the same applied to him. After dinner, I wanted to back out but the people pleaser in me couldn't do it. After all, he had driven two or more hours to meet me. He'd bought me dinner with wine and he had paid for a hotel room. I couldn't let him down. So I went with him.

As soon as I got to the room, I regretted my decision and feelings of anger and shame for myself were creeping up fast. I had sold myself short. I'll save you the details, but suffice to say that by morning, he was not happy with me. He took back the small gift that he had initially given me, told me to leave, and then he left. Fuck, what had I done to myself?

I proceeded to sit for hours in a coffee shop waiting for the stores to open so that I could get my stuff done and get the hell out of the city. I was in a daze. I felt an incredible knot in my stomach, my throat felt dry, and I was doing my best to push down all the shameful and angry emotions that were swirling around my system.

When I think about that younger self now, I give her a big energetic hug, rock her gently and whisper lovingly to her, "It's ok. It's ok. It's ok. I love you."

A few days after that encounter, having successfully pushed down the shame and anger, the man messaged me and was friendly with me again. It surprised me, but regardless I answered his message as if everything was fine. Although I continued to chat with him for a couple more weeks, I never saw him again. Let me reiterate that last part...This man lied to me about his age (by a landslide), then had the audacity to be upset in the morning, and took back the gift as well as telling me to leave....and I responded kindly to his messages after that! Really? Do you know how fucked up that is, on top of the fact that I had sold myself short in the first place? Thankfully, I finally started to see that. I had learned my lesson and made a vow to not ever sell myself short like that again. And, I haven't.

Looking at this from a different angle, I could say that this man had been a gift to me for it had finally hit me hard enough. I had let him take me to a level so low that I finally said, "Enough!" It is said that others will mirror that which is within ourselves. I had not been true to myself for years and he definitely mirrored that!

Despite having made the pact not to ever sell myself short again, I did not surrender the anger and shame at that time. I didn't know how yet. Instead I dealt with it the only way I knew how. I pushed it down where it continued to fester at a subconscious level. It was shortly after that rendezvous that I took my profile off the website. It was also around the same time that I got my second cancer diagnosis and made another promise to myself. "I am putting 100% of my focus on healing my body!" Other than staying connected with a couple of men who had become good friends, I have stopped interacting in that realm for the time being.

It's not that Ian and I are back to being monogamous. Just because society deems it inappropriate to have extramarital relationships doesn't make it wrong, in my opinion. We do what feels right for us. Having an open relationship wasn't the problem here. The problem was that I started to look for love in all the wrong places... outside of myself. The problem was that I didn't feel whole unless I was being doted on. My actions were rooted in fear - the fear of not being lovable.

Fear, one of the lowest vibrations in the whole Universe, had been festering in my body for so many years. And this fear was a form of stress that put my body in a perpetual state of survival. Was it any wonder that I had developed cancer in my body? This humbling realization had me dig deep within myself, continue to do the inner work, and find a way to truly love myself unconditionally.

Almost two years after the incident with this older man I was able to let go of this limiting belief that I was unlovable. I released it through another surrendering meditation.

I sat comfortably with soft music playing through my head phones.

I set my intention: surrender my fear of not being lovable.

I took myself back to the time when I was sitting in the coffee shop. I brought up all the emotions that I had felt that morning. I didn't hold back. I felt them thoroughly. I magnified them. I allowed myself to cry. I allowed myself to be angry. I allowed myself to feel the shame. I felt it all with gusto!

Then I told myself over and over again, "IT'S OK that I feel this fear of not being lovable. IT'S OK that I feel this fear of not being lovable. IT'S OK that I feel this fear of not being lovable. IT'S OK. IT'S OK. IT'S OK." I said this over and over again until the fear was lifted out of me into the light of love.

I don't remember how long this took, because I often do not have a concept of time while I'm in meditation. I knew when it was gone because I started to feel more relaxed in my body. I could breathe easier, and the knot in my stomach had disappeared. My jaw was unclenching, and I felt a loving, compassionate gentleness wash over me that I hadn't felt before. I bathed in this loving energy for as long as possible, knowing that this loving energy had the power to heal me.

In other words, when I became 100% okay with my belief of being unlovable, being unlovable became a nonissue. I let go of the need to be lovable, and as a result, was able to love myself. I am now able to say "no" when it's in my best interest, which is really saying "yes" to me.

CHAPTER 13

Food For Thought

F ood. I couldn't live without it, but living with it had proven to be challenging for me over the years. It was high time that I got to the bottom of my obsessions around food and learn to surrender it all. When I uncovered the root cause, it took me, yet again, all the way back to when I immigrated to Canada with my family, as a thirteen year old impressionable teenager.

Anyone who's ever been to the Netherlands knows that the bicycle is a very common mode of transportation there. With just as many bicycle paths as roads, it's an easy and affordable way to get around. This makes the Dutch, for the most part, a pretty fit bunch. Along with that, the North American fast food craze hadn't quite made its debut in Europe at that time. Healthy homemade meals were still the norm. Put these two together and the result was that obesity was almost nonexistent in those days in the Netherlands.

Canada, on the other hand, was a different story. Long, cold, and snowy winters in a vast land made it a bit of a challenge to use anything other than motorized vehicles to get around. And, of course, the North American fast food diet with large portion sizes were quite common. This is not to say that there were no healthy fit Canadians, but the rate of obesity was much higher than we had ever seen, and we were quite shocked by it, not to mention judgmental. I saw kids being bullied and ostracized at school for being obese. I heard people, including my parents, openly judging those who struggled with their weight. And although I wasn't fully aware of it at the time, I had made a subconscious observation that gaining weight meant that you were no longer lovable. Lucky for me, I participated a lot in sports, ate my mom's healthy cooking, and was at a healthy weight all the way through school.

At the age of 18, I spread my wings and left home. I was university bound. Oh, the freedom I felt! I could party as much as I wanted and stay out all night. Along with buffet style unhealthy cafeteria food, I could eat junk food anytime I wanted. Life was great! My clothes were getting a bit tighter, but I was having too much fun. I pushed down any uncomfortable feelings that I had about it. By the time I came home for Christmas, however, like a lot of other first year students, I was packing the "freshman 15". To this day,

I can still remember the words from my mom. "Jayka, what have you done?" And with those words, the feelings that arose within me was shame and fear. I felt shame for having let myself get to this state and fear that I was no longer lovable. Of course, my mom didn't mean to hurt me. She was a very loving woman who wanted the best for me and wanted me to be as healthy as possible. But those words along with my beliefs sent me for a tailspin that lasted for decades.

Not willing to give up the partying and having no choice but to eat the fatty, unhealthy cafeteria food, I came up with a solution that would give me the best of both worlds. Bulimia. Now, I knew that this wasn't healthy for me but my fear of not being lovable overrode my common sense, and I did it anyway, in secret. I managed to lose most of the weight that I'd gained but never got too thin. I maintained a healthy weight and no one ever suspected anything. I was never caught.

This sick binge/purge behaviour lasted for almost twenty years, not always severe, for I was a master at controlling myself around food. When this control snapped however, watch out! There'd be a war within me so vicious, it would put any bully to shame! I would binge on whatever I could get my hands on and then resort to purging in the toilet, which would then be followed by a bout of shame that made me feel so small and pathetic that surely no one could ever love me. I had yet again dipped so low as to do something as unhealthy and disgusting as vomiting.

Throughout it all, no one was the wiser, not even Ian. People would comment on how slim or fit my body was, even after having two babies. I was a picture of health. Somehow I always felt compassion for people who struggled with their weight, and yet I was so incredibly critical towards myself. Everything I was doing in my life at this point was to be healthy and set a good example for my kids, but this eating disorder was that shameful secret, signifying that all is not always as it seems.

As mentioned before, May of 2007 was the time that I received the devastating news of having breast cancer at the age of 38. My mother had been diagnosed with breast cancer at the age of 37 so the consensus at that time was that there was nothing I could have done to prevent this. It was hereditary. I believed that. My grandmother, who had been bulimic most of her adult life had died of metastasized esophageal cancer. My thought at the time was that although I was apparently destined to have cancer, I was going to do everything in my power to ensure that it would never come back. With that decision, I stopped being bulimic, almost cold turkey. Occasionally I regressed but those episodes were thankfully few and far between. All in all, I considered myself successfully healed and wanted to close the book on it. It wasn't until years later that I came face-to-face with the fact that I had never dealt with the root cause of why I chose to become bulimic in the first place. I opened that proverbial book again and started an inner exploration with the help of Ayahuasca.

As I alluded to before, Ayahuasca is the amazing
psychedelic plant medicine that changed my life. It was
at that first Ayahuasca retreat with Dr. Gabor Maté that
I attended, back in November of 2013, where I finally got
a bit of an inkling of just how unhealthy my relationship
with food really was. Ayahuasca gave me some insight of
the undercurrent that changed my relationship with food.
It made me realize that even though I hadn't been bulimic
for several years, the shame that I'd felt over those years was
still there, festering in my body. I came to the realization
that I needed to deal with this shame.

The first thing I did was to let go of the secret right there,
in Mexico, at the retreat. While sitting in a sharing circle
led by Gabor, a group of about 30 people who I had only
just met a few days prior, became the first people I told
about my shameful secret of bulimia. It was awful and I
cried and cried throughout my admission of it. "What must
they think of me? They must think me pathetic!" This is
what went through my head. I was filled with shame and
self judgments. Shortly after that, I made the decision that I
was going to tell as many people as it took until I could talk
about it without crying and without feeling ashamed of it.
This, to me, would signify that I was not only fully healed
from the eating disorder, but also from the shame. Little
did I know then that I still had quite a ways to go before I
would have a healthy relationship with food.

I may have stopped purging however that was all I
stopped. I made this realization while in the midst of my

surrendering journey. As it turned out, the inner control games continued to be in full force for several more years. Don't eat junk food...stay away from white bread, white rice, white pasta...don't drink the calories...only eat during these hours...only eat so much and no more...and for god's sake, never eat sugar!! That continued to be the tune of my obsessive, sick mind well beyond the time that I stopped purging. Control, control, control! It became pretty apparent to me that just because I had stopped vomiting did not mean that I was healed from bulimia. Something that I discovered more than 12 years after I stopped hovering over the toilet is that there is so much more to the disease than meets the eye.

After I completed all the Western cancer treatments in 2007, I was determined not to resort back to binging and purging. This meant I needed to tighten my reigns of control even more because, God forbid if I gained an ounce. After all, being fat would mean that I would no longer be lovable, and who would want to hang out with me then? (And to think that I considered myself healed from the eating disorder.)

Being thin without resorting to vomiting became a difficult task and sure enough, a few pounds crept on. You'd think I had gained a hundred pounds for the incredible scrutiny that I put myself under though. I remember one year, it was Easter weekend and the weather was unseasonably warm. We could actually wear shorts, something that rarely happens during that time of year in Canada. We Canadians get pretty excited when this happens.

Shorts and tank tops were dug out of the closets and half the population showed up to work the next day with a sunburn. I was no different. Out came the tank top and shorts. There was just one problem. My shorts felt tighter and the cellulite on my legs had gotten really bad (in my opinion). I was mortified. "What would people think of me? Look how ugly I am! I had gained at least 5 pounds. How could I have let myself go like that?!"

Oh, the inner dialogue was ruthless and I felt so incredibly self conscious. Did anyone else actually say anything about the weight gain? No, of course not. Did they even notice? Probably not. The only bully in this case, and every other case to do with my body image, was me.

That particular spring I came up with yet another solution to lose weight. A cleanse. That's healthy, right? I was going to tighten the reigns on my food choices even more and I'd cut out alcohol, gluten, meat, and dairy, just to kick it up a notch. On top of that, I decided to try out this new thing that I'd heard about called intermittent fasting where you only eat during a designated time of day, only consisting of a few hours. Of course, I did this in the name of healthy living, and was completely oblivious to the fact that all of it was emphasizing my already controlling, fear-based behaviour, making it all incredibly unhealthy for me. No, I'm not insinuating that cleansing and intermittent fasting is unhealthy as a rule. What I am saying is that for someone like me, who had a history with an eating disorder, it just added fuel to the already controlling behaviour and obsessive thought patterns that went through my head.

About two weeks into the intermittent fasting cleanse, I had shrunk my eating window to only six hours. In other words, I ate between noon and 6 o'clock. With that regimented eating schedule, I also shrunk my waistline and hit a number on the scale that I hadn't been able to reach since I was a teenager. Talk about being excited. My clothes felt looser, people were complimenting me, and I finally felt 'worthy'. (I put 'worthy' in quotation marks because increased feelings of worthiness based on the way we look is far removed from actual knowing that we are worthy, regardless of anything, including my size.)

Although I finished the official cleanse after 21 days, I decided to continue the intermittent fasting aspect of my diet. Eating only between noon and 6 o'clock with a couple of days of 24-hour fasts thrown in there every month for good measure. I followed this strict diet for about five years and maintained a weight of approximately 135lbs. This scheduled eating regime caused me to constantly look at the time to see if I could eat yet and learned to endure the hunger which at times would actually feel euphoric. The only time that I allowed myself to stray from this schedule was if we went out to a restaurant or were invited to our friends' homes for dinner. These occasions would create significant anxiety for me because not only did I eat past the allotted time, these meals usually consisted of unhealthy food, larger quantities and I'd often have wine with it. This anxiety would then lead me to make up for this 'unhealthy lapse' so the days following those extravagant evenings would be even more regimented where I would either not eat at all or maybe allow myself a couple of hours where I could eat a little bit. The control I had over myself was out of control. My body was a pressure cooker.

When I received the diagnosis in December of 2016, I was aware enough to realize that it was probably a good idea for me to join the masses again and start eating three meals a day. I reasoned that my body could probably use the extra fuel to help with healing. I wasn't perfect at it and still had my moments of wanting to hit the control button, but it was a start. Until I learned of water fasting and then all hell broke loose in my inner and physical world yet again!

CHAPTER 14

Water Fasting: The Last Drop In the Bucket

As mentioned earlier, I was in Mexico again at the start of our world travels in 2018. It had been a little over four years since I'd been in Yelapa for that first Ayahuasca retreat where I had gotten my first inkling that maybe I wasn't fully healed just yet from the effects of my eating disorder. I had discovered that for me the healing happened in stages and it was time to tend to the next layer.

While in Mexico, I spent my days relaxing and resting my body, and although I had decided to be more easy going with food, I was also continuing my four day water-fasting regime every three weeks, something that I had been doing for about six months. During these four days I would only drink water with lemon and/or ginger with the idea that it would starve the cancer cells.

There is reputable research behind this concept that water fasting does in fact kill cancer cells, however for someone who had a history with an eating disorder, it was definitely not a great idea. I was pretty cocky about it though, and thought I'd be fine with it. During these fasts, there were moments of complete euphoria and then there were moments that were absolutely awful. I'd barely be able to get up from lack of energy and strength, and I'd be chilled to the bone no matter what the temperature was. I'd have heart palpitations and sleepless nights and of course the hunger pangs were something else. I also became skinnier than I had ever been in my entire adult life. That became a red flag, causing the warped eating disorder thoughts to intensify even more. I felt the obsession with my weight increase and although I heard people's concerns for the fact that I was getting too skinny, I secretly loved it.

I paid a big price for following the water fasting diet. Not only was my body not healing, I'm pretty sure that it was actually making me sicker. If my body wasn't already in survival mode before, it certainly was now. And there is absolutely no healing happening of any sort when it is in survival mode. As you may have heard, being in survival mode means that the body feels threatened and therefore needs to stay alert (hence the insomnia). It needs to use its energy wisely and prepare for battle, so that things like the immune system and the digestive system are put on hold. My body was unable to absorb any nutrients. The insomnia got so bad for me that I spent hours every night staring at the ceiling. My hypothalamus (responsible for body temperature, hormone distribution, etc) was only functioning at 33% and my adrenals were completely tapped out causing me to have adrenal fatigue that took forever to heal.

More than ten years after I thought I'd stopped all aspects of my eating disorder behaviour, I was right back in the throes of it. The obsessive, unhealthy thoughts got so strong that there was finally no denying that I had a problem (sometimes it has to get worse before it gets better). The first step is always awareness of the problem. Now that I was no longer in denial of it, I knew that it was time for me to address it yet again. Thankfully, I had another Ayahuasca retreat booked and I knew that I was in good hands.

"You are worthy because you were born. Period!" This was the unforgettable message that came through for me during an Ayahuasca ceremony later that month. "It doesn't matter whether you're male or female, skinny or obese, black or white. It doesn't matter what you've done or not done. It doesn't matter where you've been or not been. It doesn't matter what the number on the scale is. You are worthy because you were born."

It wasn't until later that I truly felt the power of these words and how important it was for me to finally let go of fear and the harsh judgments I had of myself, and embrace my worthiness. In fact, this was the root cause of my obsessive behaviour around food, and exercise too, not to mention many other areas of my life.

Considering how many signs of stress appeared during the four day water fasting stints, I decided that this would be the first thing that needed to be scrapped. I realized that it was likely only making me weaker and sicker, not to mention it triggered the unhealthy obsessive thought patterns.

Along with scrapping the water fasting, I upped my meditation practice a bit and I joined a yin yoga class to learn to relax and stretch my body in a gentle way. And lastly, I practiced being more aware of my behaviour and thoughts about food throughout the day with the notion that you can't fix something that you're unaware of.

My body was starting to show some signs that things were improving, including weight gain. However, much like the time that I had put on the "freshman 15" more than thirty years before, I was feeling all kinds of heavy emotions that were triggered by the weight gain, unworthiness being at the core of all of them. This time I was determined to not crumble and go back to my old ways. I was going to rise above it all.

I quickly realized that this wasn't going to happen overnight. These thoughts were sneaky and tended to be persistent especially at the beginning, but I was just going to have to be more persistent in my quest to let them go.

The minute I became aware of the unworthy thoughts, I would rise above them. I did this by telling myself that they weren't real; they were just an interesting point of view. It was one of many tools that I had learned from a few Access Consciousness courses that I had taken and they served me well.

I learned that the awareness comes from the observer. Who is the observer? Your higher self, your soul. Your soul observes the ego and all the thoughts and behaviours that happen throughout the day. The soul exists at a high vibration so when I would consciously rise up to that vibration, I would feel calmer, more loving and more allowing. And of course the idea was to function from my soul's perspective as much as I possibly could. But like I said before, that darn ego of mine was sneaky and more often than not, before I knew it, I was back in the thralls of negative thoughts. As frustrating as it was, I was not giving up. There was just too much at stake. I was going to master that ego of mine no matter what it took!

At this point, I had not come to the realization yet that it would be very beneficial for me to befriend my ego. Ever hear of the phrase "What you resist, persists"? Apparently that applies to the ego as well. But, I wasn't there yet. Instead, I was prepared to hunt the ego down and kill it!

Although there was some progress with the 'interesting point of view' tool or 'IPOV' as they like to call it in the world of Access, my patience was tested. I was no quitter though and thoughts like "I will prevail" kept me going.

And prevail I did. As I continued to focus on self love, I became more and more relaxed with food. As a matter of fact, about a year later, I had my pH tested at a holistic clinic in Thailand and it showed that my body was no longer acidic. This was huge and something that I had strived for in the past. When I became vegan two years prior, it was because I wanted to give my body mostly alkaline food (animal products are acidic), but no matter what I tried back then, I could not get my pH levels out of the acidic zone. And considering that disease thrives in acidic bodies, this was a serious concern. So there I was in Asia, where it was definitely more challenging to eat healthy, and I indulged quite a bit more than ever before with the conscious decision to relax and enjoy all the food that I ate. I did this while also feeling the love for my body, and voilà, my body was loved, relaxed, and able to absorb the nutrients, which in turn balanced my pH level, providing my body with an environment that was conducive for healing.

As I think back to those years where my mind was filled with obsessive controlling thoughts and beliefs, I wonder how I never clued in to the insanity of it all. In fact, I often promoted the intermittent fasting and the water fasting diets to others. I would tell anyone who'd listen how amazing those diets were and how healthy it was for our bodies, especially because the fasting hours would also starve any possible cancer cells that may be floating around in your body. I believed it was a surefire way that I would not ever be diagnosed with cancer again. Obviously, that didn't work out quite how I had thought it would. I did that all for a couple of pounds that no one but myself was aware of, and all because I deemed myself unlovable if those extra pounds made their way onto my ass. Oh, if only I knew then what I know now. It would have saved me a lot of heart ache. However, on the flip side, it would have also prevented me from having the amazing opportunity of growth that I ultimately experienced.

Here is another surrendering meditation that helped me through this.

I sat comfortably with my eyes closed and soft music playing into my head phones.

I set my intention: surrender my belief that being overweight means you're unlovable.

I brought up all the emotions that were attached to the belief that being overweight meant I was unlovable. I didn't hold back. I imagined myself with an extra 100 pounds and felt the fear intensify. I magnified it even more. The tears streamed down my face. I allowed myself to feel shame. I allowed myself to feel guilt. I allowed myself to feel the fear. I felt it all with gusto!

Then, I told myself over and over again, "IT'S OK that I feel this fear of not being lovable. IT'S OK that I feel this fear of not being lovable. IT'S OK that I feel this fear of not being lovable. IT'S OK. IT'S OK. IT'S OK." I said this over and over again until the fear was lifted out of me into the light of love. I knew when it was gone because I started to feel more relaxed in my body. I could breathe easier, and the knot in my stomach had disappeared. I no longer had a lump in my throat. I felt a loving, compassionate gentleness wash over me that I hadn't felt earlier. I bathed in this loving energy for as long as possible, knowing that this loving energy had the power to heal me.

In other words, when I became 100% okay with my fear of being unlovable, it became a nonissue and I was okay with it. I realized that I had not loved myself all these years and that this was the real issue. This surrendering meditation allowed me to finally love myself unconditionally.

Are there moments that I'm tempted to go back to my old behaviours? Yes. And when I am, I know I've lost touch with who I am for a moment. Those moments never last very long before I remember who I AM, and I tune into her once again...

I AM LOVE

I AM so grateful that this beautiful worthy woman allows me to take her into my arms and tell her to relax, to let go, that everything is ok. When this controlling sick behaviour tries to creep up, I hold her gently and keep telling her, "It's ok. It's ok. It's ok." I remind her daily that she's worthy, regardless of the number on the scale or what she sees in the mirror. I interject her almost immediately when she starts to scrutinize herself, continually telling her that it's ok. I now cheer her on when she chooses to eat breakfast, lunch and dinner, which happens almost daily now. I AM the LOVE that is her true essence. I AM the LOVE that is so powerful it keeps her immune system strong, allowing her body to relax and absorb all the nutrients. It balances her hormones; it helps her sleep through the night; it brings her inner peace; it brings her inner joy. This is the Love that continually heals her body. Love heals.

CHAPTER 15

The Poverty Complex

The first time that I got an inkling about exactly how much of a stressful impact money had on my body was at that first Ayahuasca retreat in Mexico in 2013. Ayahuasca had helped me successfully release all kinds of pent up energy in several areas of my life except in relation to money.

It seemed that I was stuck, in a big way. There was actual physical pain in my body during ceremony that was so strong that it persevered beyond the six hours of that ceremony and started up again the following day. This physical pain represented the fear that I would end up broke and homeless. Thankfully, I was under the guidance of a beautiful woman, Shannon, who had a lot of experience and knowledge with Ayahuasca. She sat with me for hours that following day and gently comforted me as shameful memories came to the surface that I was apparently not ready to deal with. Memories of theft...

I started working as a waitress and bartender during the summers when I was nineteen. I was young, impressionable, and irresponsible. It was a pretty common practice back then for the bartenders and waiters to steal from the establishment where I worked, and I joined in without giving it much thought. I had never really stolen before but for whatever reason, I got caught up in this and didn't fully realize the seriousness of it until later.

We would steal by not keying in certain items into the computer as we served them, or we'd use the same bill more than once while pocketing the money. Sometimes we'd hide liquor in a garbage bag during a banquet and sneak it out at the end of our shift, although I rarely joined in on that. I didn't really like hard liquor. It didn't add up to loads of money, but that's not the point. It was still theft.

After a few years of this, I was caught when I served a secret shopper. He ordered a liqueur which I actually punched into the computer, but before I had a chance to make it, he stopped me and said that he'd changed his mind and wanted a different, more expensive liqueur. I served it to him but forgot to void the initial liqueur and replace it with the other. He left cash on the table without asking for the bill, and left. I had been set up, but that's what they do. The irony was that I had actually forgotten to make the correction, so I didn't do it deliberately. The next day I was called into my boss' office. My heart was pounding as I felt my temperature rising while I quietly sat there holding my breath. I was a nervous wreck. Luckily, I was given the benefit of the doubt when I told them that I'd forgotten to change it in the computer. My boss believed me and I got to keep my job. Phew!

This experience shook me up enough to realize that what I had been doing was definitely not kosher. Yes, I was stressed about money, but that's no reason to steal. I stopped stealing out of fear of getting caught again, but also because my conscience prevented me from ever doing it again. As a matter of fact, I swung the other way and became quite obsessed about ensuring that everything was punched into the computer as it should be. I felt shame and guilt whenever I thought of it. I actually made a couple of donations in an attempt to balance out the energy of it but the guilt was still there, festering in my body. Secrets will eat you up.

There I was, more than twenty years later, at the Ayahuasca retreat, unable to release this heavy fearful energy of money. And although I had no idea how, I knew how important it was for me to find allowance for my behaviour and shine a light onto this fear around money, and learn to surrender it all. That was more than six years ago and although I've come a long way and improved leaps and bounds with my fears around money, I feel that there's still more room for improvement. Just ask Ian.

Where did this fear come from? This poverty complex that I had struggled with? There was even a fear of becoming homeless. How could that be? I'd come from a middle class family. I'd not ever gone hungry and had always had a roof over my head....what gives? Well, there are a couple of options that I've looked into, one has to do with past lives and the other is the intergenerational factor. Both seemed to have impacted me in this lifetime.

About three years ago, I booked a past life session purely out of curiosity. I had not considered a link between my current life and any past lives and how that link might impact me today, but I was open to it. The past life that I visited during that session was that of a homeless man who was illiterate, unable to find work, ridiculed by society, and eventually beaten to death. It was a life of fear, hunger, sadness, and disempowerment. I came out of that session quite disappointed for I had hoped to visit a much more exciting and empowered life. However, as I was reminded by Dave, the practitioner, we don't learn as much from the seemingly more successful lives. I was also told to pay attention over the next few weeks because synchronicities may happen with regard to this past life session and if that were to happen, he would be interested in hearing about it.

As luck would have it, synchronicity did in fact come into play a couple of weeks after the session. I had just dropped off my daughter at a week long Ayahuasca retreat in Nelson, British Columbia, about a thousand kilometres from our home. Instead of driving back, I decided to hang out in the beautiful Kootenay area by myself until her retreat was finished. With my luggage, a cooler, and a lawn chair in the trunk, I set off to explore.

While having a picnic lunch by Kootenay Lake in Nelson, I was greeted by a clean cut man who was walking his bicycle. Upon acknowledging him, he decided that this was an invitation and he sat down beside me. His name was Terrence and he was homeless. Of course this made me sit up and take note. He was a lovely man who proceeded to talk my ear off for about two hours while I shared my lunch with him. I could barely get a word in edgewise, but I suspected that he didn't often have an audience and I was happy to sit and listen to him.

The story of his childhood was heartbreaking. Learning of his lack of family roots combined with his mental health struggles, I could feel compassion and understand that these were the core reasons for his homeless situation. He'd been homeless for decades, but regardless, he seemed to thrive in his own way. He was proud to tell me that he no longer slept on the ground, but instead lived in an old boat under the dock. "It's illegal but the cops like me, so they don't bother me," he assured me. He was so proud of his humble abode that he insisted on showing me. I felt quite safe with him so I agreed, after all we were in a public place. His boat did not have a cover so I could just imagine how cold it must be for him during the winter time, but he assured me that he had lots of blankets and warm clothing to keep him toasty. He grabbed a crystal from the dash and presented it to me as a gift. I was very touched.

Terrence was clean cut and dressed nicely because he had just returned from volunteering at the soup kitchen where he was also able to get cleaned up. This organization often gave him food and clothing to take along with him. Terrence was a spiritual man and was quite excited to show me the scarf that they had given him that morning. "They gave me this orange silk scarf that is obviously meant for a woman," he told me, "so I wasn't sure what the hell I was supposed to do with it. It's definitely not going to keep me warm, that's for sure!" He continued. And then he gave me a big smile, "Now I know that I'm meant to give you this scarf. It's orange, your Dutch national colour!" And with that, he gifted me the beautiful scarf.

In this short amount of time, a man who seemingly had nothing, proceeded to give me two gifts. I was so touched; he was a very special soul. When he proclaimed his love for me and wanted me to have his children I knew that it was time to pack up my stuff and hit the road. He had told me earlier that blueberries were his favourite fruit and that before our picnic, he hadn't had them for years. So I gave him the Costco sized container of blueberries along with a big hug and kiss on the cheek.

I called Dave a couple of weeks later to tell him about my interactions with Terrence and at precisely the moment that I told Dave about giving Terrence a hug and kiss, I realized that I had in that moment embraced the homeless man within me and let go of the resistance. I will never forget Terrence. He showed me that even when you're homeless, you can thrive as a human being. Although I would still struggle with money in the years to come, thanks to Terrence, I was able to let go of the fear of becoming homeless.

That was an example of past life baggage being healed. Here is an example of intergenerational baggage.

Dr. Gabor Maté had spoken of intergenerational issues and it all resonated with me. I come from generations of farmers on both sides of the family where feast or famine was the norm for centuries. Even when they were feasting, there was always the underlying fear of when the so-called famine would hit, so saving up for a rainy day was of course a responsible way to counter this. However, I now realize that the energy around saving up for a rainy day is that of fear. That energy of fear was passed down all the way to me. My parents, especially my father, played a big role in continuing this intergenerational pattern. My parents were both born during World War Two when everything was rationed. Their parents also had lived through World War One as well as the depression. As I mentioned previously, children are like sponges and take on the beliefs of those who raise them. Is it any wonder that my parents had a fearful relationship with money?

Despite these fears, my father had done quite well on a financial level in that he had money in the bank, but it consumed him. He was obsessed with it, in my opinion. Money was his favourite topic of conversation and I imagine that he thought about it all the time. In February of 2018, my father drove himself to the hospital, a place that he had given a wide berth ever since my mother passed away. My father had Parkinson's and was afraid that if he went to the doctor that he would lose his licence. He was feeling so sick, however, that he knew that it couldn't be avoided. Sure enough, the doctor took one look at him and took away his licence. The doctor also wouldn't let him go home. He was in such bad shape that he was forced to go into a senior's home. He also learned that he'd had blood poisoning and bladder cancer. It was a lot to absorb. For someone who needed control, he had lost most of it in one fell swoop. The one area of control that he still had left though was that of money.

Whenever I become aware that the fear around money has come up, and it still does occasionally. I surrender immediately. I've worked on this topic often enough that I don't even need to go into a meditation. I simply tell myself quietly, or in my head, it's okay that I'm afraid of becoming bankrupt, repeating as often as needed while allowing the fearful emotions to come up so I can feel the discomfort fully. Usually, within seconds I feel them dissipating and I'm once again relaxed, in tune with my true essence.

CHAPTER 16

Speak Up!

I'm not 100% at ease with coming out and sharing my innermost secrets that I've written about in this book. To say writing about it has created vulnerability within me is a definite understatement. I guess it's not every day that someone voluntarily admits to theft, her struggles with an eating disorder, or her unconventional bedroom activities. How will people react? Will my friends ditch me? Am I going to be an outcast?

I came clean to Ian and our two adult children without much drama, thanks to their unconditional love for me... but, what about the people outside my little family? There was only one way to find out. I decided to test it out on a couple of close friends. Yep, I know. I was still playing it safe by choosing friends who likely wouldn't reject me, but it was a start.

Then, my friend suggested I share with two women I had met only once before, two years prior. Yikes! Nothing like getting thrown to the wolves, although I knew that my friend's intention was filled with love by helping me take it to the next level.

"Alright then, no time like the present," and with that, I told them. The sky didn't come falling down. Nothing blew up in my face. They didn't run for the hills. In fact, they were still hanging out with me and still smiling without throwing even an ounce of judgment my way. Ok, maybe this won't make a complete pariah out of me after all.

Since that weekend, I have shared my secrets with several other people, both close friends as well as new acquaintances, and I started to notice a pattern. As I was showing my vulnerability by sharing my secrets, I inadvertently opened up a door for them to share secrets of their own that brought them regret and shame. From admitting to stealing wine from a church as a teenager, to shoplifting, to agreeing to have sex because my friend also couldn't say no, it seemed that I wasn't the only one who had strayed beyond what is deemed as acceptable behaviour at one point or another. One gal even admitted to not ever having told her secret to anyone until she shared it with me. How powerful is that? It reminded me of the Me Too movement. We are not alone in this and talking about it is an important step in the healing journey.

More often than not, secrets have shame and regret

attached to them. For that reason, secrets cause our energy to contract. Contracted energy is heavy and gets stuck, causing dis-ease in our bodies which of course leads to disease. Expansion allows energy to flow freely throughout our bodies keeping it healthy and strong. As I mentioned previously, my sister-in-law never spoke truer words than when she said, "Secrets will eat you up" and like I said, "So will cancer."

This is where I pass the baton over to you and ask you to put the magnifying glass on yourself with self-compassion and honesty. Have there been times in your life that you've secretly done things that you regret and feel ashamed of? Perhaps you've held onto those secrets for decades. Maybe you assume that it's been so long that you've moved on and are done with it. May I remind you that my days of stealing happened thirty years ago and was still festering in my body. How did I know that it was still festering? Because whenever I thought about it, I felt regret, guilt and shame creeping up. Let me tell you from experience, ignoring them does not make them go away. Instead they fester, possibly keeping you from being as healthy as you could be.

For me, surrendering these secrets as well as speaking up for myself in other areas of my life has healed my body in more ways than one. I didn't just have cancer in my body. I also had other conditions, one being hypothyroidism, a condition that has become all too common, especially among women. I was diagnosed with this shortly after getting the recurring cancer diagnosis. I was told that thyroid problems increase a woman's chance for developing breast cancer four-fold so I likely had thyroid problems for years without having a clue. Not something that anyone wants to hear. Nor do we want to hear that it's likely a life-long condition. Thankfully, I decided not to believe the latter. It may be a life-long condition for some, but I was going to get to the bottom of it and considered it only a temporary condition.

I love the work of Dr. Joe Dispenza. He has a couple of meditations that focus on the energy centres (chakras) that I did on a daily basis for several months. These meditations had me moving the energy from the first energy centre (root chakra) all the way up through the rest of my energy centres and out my crown (top of my head). Seems easy enough, except I always noticed that the energy would get stuck in my throat chakra. I would literally start coughing and feel the need to swallow excessively. Over time, my throat chakra slowly started to relax.

Incidentally, I had been decreasing my thyroid medications on a regular basis over the past year or so. I went off the medications completely at the beginning of June, 2019. However, a few symptoms reappeared letting me know that my body wasn't 100% healed yet. As disappointing as that was, I'm also all about listening to my body. Therefore, I started taking a small dose of the medicine again, literally, only 1/8 of a pill (I couldn't even cut the pill that small so I bit a quarter in half).

It's interesting that when I wrote hypothyroidism into the search engine, the first article that came up was called: Hypothyroidism: A Silent Epidemic. Of course, I interpreted that literally where hypothyroidism is a symptom of being silent instead of speaking up for yourself. Apparently, that's not what the author of the article meant. The author called it silent because so many of the symptoms mimic other health issues and the thyroid is often overlooked or not tested accurately. Other articles listed all kinds of suggestions that could possibly help hypothyroidism along with medication, such as a variety of supplements, diet changes, etc. But nowhere did it say anything about its connection to the throat chakra. The thyroid is located in the throat, a chakra that functions as the voice of our body. Wouldn't it make sense to explore that?

If there is, in fact, an epidemic of thyroid problems in the world right now, especially in the female population, what does that say about our behaviour? It speaks volumes doesn't it? I'd say it's our body telling us in no uncertain terms that this silent behaviour is not benefitting us in the least and that it's high time to reassess. Is it easy? Absolutely not. In fact, it's incredibly difficult to step up and be heard when you've avoided it for decades. After all, isn't that the reason that we've avoided it in the first place? But look at the huge price that we're paying by staying in our comfort zone. Ironically, this comfort zone is not all that comfortable after all. All it is doing is putting us in a state of dis-ease. Let's step up, not just for ourselves, but also for future generations. Considering our children tend to mimic us, let's ensure that they're mimicking empowered behaviour. Let's set an example and show them that being willing to be uncomfortable and vulnerable is a sign of strength of which the pay-off is exponential. The more you do it, the more confident you'll become and the more comfortable you'll eventually be with yourself. Who knows, you may even inspire your friends to do the same. Let's be trail blazers together.

If I've piqued your interest, my suggestion is to set yourself up for success. Before you bare your soul, prepare yourself for a meditation with an intention, asking for clarity and ease with this task. Of course, unconditional love and compassion for yourself always goes without saying. While in meditation, stay with the emotions that arise in regard to the situation at hand, the one that you've been silent about, whether it be a shameful secret or an occasion where you've just not had the courage to speak up for yourself.

Be prepared to feel resistance and stay with the uncomfortable emotions until they lighten up. Continually assure yourself by saying, "It's okay to feel this discomfort." Do this until it lightens up and you feel the compassionate love. Bathe in this love while also expanding out your energy and visualize yourself having spoken your truth, as if it has already happened. Along with that, reach for the emotions that you would feel as if it had already happened. Would you feel relief? Gratitude? Freedom? Empowered? Then, go ahead and feel exactly that. Stay in that expansive, feel good space for as long as you can. It may be beneficial to do the latter feel good part of this meditation a few times to really let it become you.

Then, when you're ready, it's show time. Find the courage within you to actually do this. (Keep in mind that if there's a history of abuse in your life and your safety is at risk, this does not apply to you. In that case, you need to seek help and remove yourself from that relationship.)

It may be beneficial for you to write down some pointers of what you want to say, or you can trust that whatever needs to be said will come out perfectly on its own accord.

Determine when and where you're going to speak your truth. Find a location where there'll not be any distractions or interruptions and give yourself ample time. I've found that a parked car on an isolated parking lot is a great place to have deep conversations. Going on a walk together in nature or sitting in a private spot by a lake or river are also great options. Do whatever will work for you. And finally, ensure that you are speaking from your own perspective, avoiding accusations and finger pointing, remembering all the while that you are not a victim here. You chose to be silent and now you're choosing to speak up for yourself. Congratulations! This is your moment of truth. Embrace it.

As I write these encouraging words to you, I've become even more aware of the importance that I tap into the power of speaking up for myself in regard to my father. I've yet to do it. The thought of it makes me very uncomfortable. Will I have the courage? Will it completely heal my thyroid when I do?

CHAPTER 17

Standing In My Power With My Father

Despite the fact that my father and I had come a long way in our relationship and everything was good on the surface, the undercurrents were still a bit choppy. My father liked to play mind games and like I mentioned before, he thrived on control, specifically with money. I had never asked my father for money, mainly because I just wasn't comfortable doing it. And I had a fear of rejection in that area as well.

Because his relationship with money had always been quite OCD in my opinion, I avoided the topic like the plague. However, when he told me during the spring of 2017 how he had given my brother a significant loan a few years earlier to help set up his business, I decided that I would gather up the courage and ask my father for a loan as well. I would never have considered it except that I was several months into my holistic treatment protocol for cancer and the medical bills were piling up. Being that he had helped my brother, I felt somewhat confident that he would be willing to help me out as well. But unfortunately, it seemed that I was wrong. I was once again rejected.

I was disappointed, but it was not totally unexpected. I was proud of myself for having found the courage to ask him. In the end it all worked out because we sold our home, most of our belongings, payed off the medical bills, and were able to travel for fifteen months on top of that. My father did call me later and told me that he would make some changes to the will so that there was extra money to cover the cost of my treatments. So it wasn't a complete rejection, but after his passing I became aware that he had later changed it, and taken it out. Being unaware of this at the time, I had come to terms with my father's decision, but learned a few months later that he had helped his daughter-in-law pay for a very expensive quantum energy machine that helped heal her from Lyme disease.

While I was happy that they'd found a way to cure this horrific disease, at the same time I was very hurt. My father had told me that he did not have any liquidated money to give me which was obviously not true. My father was known to show his love, respect, and appreciation to others with money. Apparently he felt none of that towards me. Once again, the feeling of rejection reared its ugly head. I felt small, worthless, and unwanted.

To top it off, while visiting my father the following summer I learned that there was more that he hadn't told me. We went to a Thai restaurant for lunch where all the tables were taken and we needed to wait. There was an older couple sitting at a six-top who were kind enough to invite us over and let us join them at their table. My father monopolized the conversation and talked a lot about his health and how he was helping his daughter-in-law with financing a medical degree. I just about fell off my chair with shock! He was financing what? Was he trying to hurt me on purpose?

My nervous system went into overdrive with jitteriness but I kept my shock and despair to myself and covered it up with a smile, albeit quivery. When it came time to pay the bill, my father turned to me and said, "Are you going to pay for lunch? You've got lots of money right? You just sold your house." Talk about pouring a bucket of salt onto the wound. I felt the tears rise up in my throat yet again, but managed to keep it together, smile and all. With a "Yes, I've got it", I got up and paid for the bill.

I don't know if my father realized just how much he hurt me but I started to realize more and more that our relationship was unfortunately very superficial. Yes, we were on speaking terms but we were definitely not speaking the same language. It is possible that my father had an inkling of how I felt though because he admitted to me later that week that the reason he didn't want to help me financially was because he didn't believe in my choices of modalities.

I briefly attempted to explain to him how I was being guided by my inner wisdom on this healing journey, but it went onto deaf ears. Instead, he tried to convince me to buy the same quantum energy machine that he'd bought for his daughter-in-law. There was one problem though. I knew intuitively that this machine wasn't meant for me. I was inspired to follow my own specific path and it was important to me to continue on that path. Thankfully my inner people pleaser stayed out of the picture for once and I was strong enough in my conviction that I didn't sway. Much like what I had told the surgeon the previous year, I told my father that I wasn't interested in it at that time.

The fact that my father didn't believe in me or my inner wisdom was something else for me to process. All in all it had been a pretty stressful week that had brought up all kinds of shit for me to let go of one way or another.

I dug deep for the coming year to let go of this rejection energy that I felt so strongly with regard to my father. I called him on a few occasions throughout the year which would only trigger these feelings more. It seemed as if I was getting nowhere with this. I felt stuck. The last time I spoke with my father before visiting him for his 80th birthday during the spring of 2019 was a doozy. I remember being in Vietnam on a gorgeous beach with Ian. I had spoken with my father that morning and was still feeling quite vulnerable while on the beach. Once again, my father was playing mind games and the rejection devastated me.

I decided to go into the sea to cool off in more ways than one. Ian wasn't interested in joining me. I went in alone while he stayed on the beach. I was surrounded by couples who were enjoying the water together. I then saw Ian get up and walk toward the water and thought to myself, "Awesome, he's going to join me." But he didn't. He swam in the opposite direction. Well, if that didn't trigger more rejection within me. It likely wouldn't have bothered me at all except that I was already in a vulnerable state.

By this time I had taught myself to stop stuffing down emotions. But here I was, in a public area, surrounded by people. It was definitely not an ideal place to fall apart. However, that didn't seem to matter. The feelings of rejection had flooded to the surface along with the tears. With the comfort of knowing that no one knew me there anyway and very few of them spoke English, I was a blubbering mess while telling Ian how hurt I was. Of course, he didn't purposely reject me. Ian is a very kind and loving man, but he was getting frustrated with me.

"You spoke with your dad this morning, didn't you?" he asked. "And I'm the one that gets blamed!" I didn't mean for Ian to feel blamed and I was well aware that my father had been the trigger, but I needed to talk it out instead of stuff it down, and Ian was my sounding board. Ian deserves a medal for standing by my side while I surrendered all my baggage, day in and day out.

I knew it was high time that I focus on letting go of this

feeling of rejection. It was time that I embraced the fact that I was whole, and that which is whole cannot be rejected. The other aspect that I needed to look at was my own vibration towards my father. I remembered how I had cleaned up my end of our energetic cord five years prior by allowing him to be who he was without judgments, and how that caused my father to lower his defences and accept my offer of reconnection. It made me wonder...had I muddled up my end of this energetic cord again? Was that why he was treating me this way? After all, it takes two to tango. The answer was a resounding YES. I had let my judgments creep back in along with resentment and neediness. It was time that I focused on loving my father unconditionally along with loving myself and knowing that regardless of how I had been treated, I am whole.

This became my focus in meditation to prepare myself for my visit with my father later that spring.

I laid comfortably with my eyes closed and soft music playing into my head phones.

I set my intention: surrender my fear of rejection by my father.

I brought up all the emotions that were attached to the beliefs of being unworthy and unlovable. I didn't hold back. I felt it thoroughly. I magnified it. As always, it was uncomfortable, but I persevered. I allowed myself to cry, a lot. I allowed myself to feel the sadness. I allowed myself to feel anger. I allowed myself to feel the fear. I felt it all with gusto!

Then, I told myself over and over again, "IT'S OK that I feel this fear of not being lovable. IT'S OK that I feel this fear of not being lovable. IT'S OK that I feel this fear of not being lovable. IT'S OK. IT'S OK. IT'S OK." I said this over and over again until the fear was lifted out of me into the light of love. I knew when it was gone because I started to feel more relaxed in my body. I could breathe easier, and the knot in my stomach had disappeared. My throat no longer felt constricted. I felt a loving, compassionate gentleness wash over me that I hadn't felt earlier. I bathed in this loving energy for as long as possible, knowing that this loving energy had the power to heal me.

In other words, when I became 100% okay with my fear of being unlovable, it became a nonissue and I was okay with it. I once again realized that I had not loved myself all these years and that this was the real issue. This surrendering meditation allowed for me to love my father unconditionally as well as finally know my self-worth. I embodied love.

CHAPTER 18

The Last Few Months With My Father

Ian was concerned about me going to New Brunswick to visit my father for his birthday. He didn't want a repeat of my last visit with him. I had come so far with my emotional healing that he didn't want me to lose ground. I felt confident that all would be well. I embodied worthiness. My father wouldn't be able to touch that with a ten foot pole! My brother, Roelof, made plans to fly in as well, giving Ian peace of mind. Roelof and I have always had a good bond and he would make sure that the visit went smoothly. Little did we know that one simple question that Roelof asked ended up having a ripple effect that caused me to rock the boat that week, something that I was finally feeling courageous enough to do.

As Roelof and I were driving from the airport to my father's place, Roelof said, "Did you know that dad believes that you and Ian are broke?"

"What? We're not broke!" was my shocked reply. "What makes him think that? We made sure to keep money aside after our travels to get us set up for our next chapter, and we still own a house that we rent out." Knowing that my father had lots of judgments for those who are irresponsible with money, I knew that if he believed that we were broke, he would be filled with those same judgments towards Ian and me. I just shook my head. I'm not sure how he came to this conclusion, but it seemed that he was determined to continue his mind games with me.

The following day was Sunday, the day of my father's birthday party. Thirteen people had been invited. There would be dinner, birthday cake, and of course, a few presents. I started my day off with a meditation as I always did. Sometimes, during these meditations, I receive messages from my higher self. This was one of those times. The message came through loud and clear. "PAY FOR THE BIRTHDAY DINNER." What? Seriously? That could be $500 or more!

Again I heard, "PAY FOR THE BIRTHDAY DINNER." Since I had long since learned to listen to these messages, I did exactly that. Dinner would be my birthday present to my father, regardless of how much it would cost.

Later that day, at the restaurant, I slipped out half way through dinner and paid the bill. Since there had been no alcohol served, it was just dinner and tea. The bill ended up being just over $200. Wow. I had been totally prepared to pay at least $500. I couldn't believe it. It still makes me smile as I think about that moment.

My father became aware that I had paid for dinner a little later on but didn't say anything about it to me. I knew that he definitely hadn't expected it. Did I mention that this birthday dinner was at the exact same Thai restaurant where my father and I had gone the previous summer when he suggested that I pay for lunch, because I'd sold my house and had lots of money? It seemed we had come full circle.

Roelof and I drove my father back to the senior's lodge that evening and as we said our goodbyes, my father said to Roelof, "Thank you for the great gift, and please make sure that you tell Stacy too how much I appreciate the gift." He spoke not a word to me about my gift. There was no acknowledgement whatsoever that he knew that I'd paid for the birthday dinner. He had, in fact, rejected it. Why was I still letting myself be surprised by his mind games? I should have been used to it by now. But something felt different than before. I was aware of the rejection, and I didn't feel affected by it at all. As a matter of fact, I felt pretty light. I was a little in awe of it... those surrendering meditations really do work.

That night, as I laid in bed, a feeling of complete expanded ecstasy overcame me. I was lying there, glowing and grinning from ear to ear, feeling at one with my beautiful soul, embodying the Love. It was absolutely amazing!

Something huge had shifted within me. Not just the energy of rejection but also the fearful energy of money had shifted. I felt nothing but complete freedom. Hallelujah!

All these years I had bent over backwards to avoid rejection and get people to love me, and all I needed to do was look within and nurture my inner love. It turns out that I had been the biggest source of my own rejection. Once I embodied love, rejection from others, including my father, became a non-issue.

The rest of the week with my father went amazingly well. I felt more like the witness of the interactions with him, instead of being caught up in them. He never did acknowledge, nor thank me for my birthday gift, and that's ok. I was just so grateful for the healing that had happened within me.

Quite innocently, I assumed that the relationship between my father and I couldn't get any better than this. After all, I had finally freed myself of that stubborn rejection energy. Well, it appeared that my higher self, my inner being, had an even more expansive vision for me... go figure. This vision came through as a message in meditation about six weeks later.

"Tell dad…" I instantly knew what those two words implied. Since this message didn't come through overly loud, I quickly pushed it aside with a "Are you kidding me? No way! That's not happening! There's a reason I haven't given him the details of my healing journey. Never mind that he's practically on his death bed. I can't do this to him now! I love him!"

As you can see, this was definitely not something I had any interest in doing, to say the least. Goes to show that there were layers within this fear of rejection paradigm. This was a leap I thought I wasn't ready for.

Several days passed and the message came through again, this time with a bit more oomph, "TELL DAD...".
I started sobbing, right then and there, while still in meditation. "Please don't ask this of me. I can't do this!"

"Yes, you can do it. It's time that you completely balance the energies between the two of you. It's ok; your dad will be ok." This inner dialogue had my nervous system going into a tizzy!

Fuck! "Don't you know I hate confrontation, especially with dad?" But the writing was on the wall. I needed to do this. Yes, I could have continued to ignore this message and it probably would have left my energy field eventually, but at what expense? In the large scope of evolution, this was possibly going to be like a rocket for my soul's evolution. It was an opportunity to finally balance out the energies between us after fifty years...in this lifetime...never mind all the other lifetimes that we've hung out together. Ok, that's pretty huge.

Meanwhile, I knew there would be a big sacrifice that I'd have to make, because this wouldn't go over well at all. My father would hopefully hear me out, then he'd go into the offence. He'd likely write me out of his will, and probably wouldn't ever want to talk to me again.

I was willing to sacrifice it all for the greater good.

As I spoke to him over the phone, I felt calm, as if it wasn't me who was speaking. The only time that a sob came up was when I talked about my eating disorder that was triggered by his judgments.

My father did hear me out (for the most part) and then charged in his usual way. "You're brainwashed" was his first retaliation. "I studied this in the army. I know about this. You're brainwashed." he concluded.

Brainwashed…that's an interesting label. As I thought about it, that label was quite fitting for my old self - the self that believed lies such as I'm not enough, I'm unworthy, I'm unlovable, I'm unimportant, etc. But I kept those thoughts to myself, not wanting to turn this into a match and make it any more uncomfortable than it already was. He continued to lash out at me for a bit longer. I told him that despite all of it, I loved him and I was grateful for him, and that I did this to balance the energies between us.

He, of course, did not agree nor understand. I left the ball in his court with, "I won't contact you, but if you'd like to talk to me again, and I hope that you do, please call me." And I said goodbye. I had managed to keep it together for the most part throughout the conversation but the moment

I hung up, I broke down and sobbed. That conversation was definitely up there with being one of the most difficult things I'd ever done in my life. I was in a daze for the rest of the day, just going through the motions, feeling numb.

I woke up the next morning and remembered it almost instantaneously. I felt sick about it and doubt had started to creep in. Maybe I had misunderstood the message in my meditation. What had I done? My father had told me not to bother seeing him on his death bed with apologies. So there was no turning back. What was done, was done. I just had to live with it now. I sent a group message out to my two brothers and sisters-in-law to get them up to speed, to which one brother responsed, "Well, that was stupid." Thankfully, another response was much more loving.

Feeling raw with emotions, I grabbed the dog and took off into nature. Surrounded by magnificent trees, I instantly felt calmer. I took some deep breaths and opened up my entire body to the Universal love, and then it was as if there were all of a sudden a thousand suns shining down on earth. Everything looked magnificently bright! I felt incredible love for everything. I felt my father's love all around me while being fully aware that it was the love of my father's soul that I felt and not his ego. Of course! My father's soul is part of the unconditional love of the Universe. I was tapped into the Universal love myself, enabling me to feel his soul's love. It was amazing. It was incredible. When I arrived home, I thought about my brothers and sisters-in-law, thinking that they must be quite angry with me as well, and all I felt from them was also beautiful loving energy. I remained in total bliss that entire day, vibrating on a magnificent high. It was so expansive, I could almost imagine my soul high-fiving my father's soul.

I thanked my higher self for having given me this difficult task. I was so grateful for this incredible enlightening day that it removed all the doubt that I had about having had that conversation with my father.

All was well then, right? Not quite. The next day, I had come off that blissful high and felt the doubt creep in again, making me realize that this would be a rollercoaster ride for the time being and to surrender to all of it, the highs, the lows, and everything in between.

So, I meditated.

I laid comfortably with my eyes closed and soft music playing into my head phones.

I set my intention: surrender the belief that I should not have called my father.

I brought up all the emotions that were attached to this belief. I didn't hold back. I felt it thoroughly. I magnified it. As always, it was uncomfortable but I persevered. I allowed myself to cry, a lot. I allowed myself to feel the regret. I allowed myself to feel doubt. I allowed myself to feel despair. As usual, I felt it all with gusto.

Then, I told myself over and over again, "IT'S OK that I feel doubt and despair. IT'S OK that I feel doubt and despair. IT'S OK that I feel doubt and despair. IT'S OK. IT'S OK. IT'S OK." I said this over and over again until the doubt and despair was lifted out of me into the light of love. I knew when it was gone, because I started to feel more relaxed in my body, and I could breathe easier. The knot in my stomach had disappeared and my throat no longer felt constricted. I felt a loving, compassionate gentleness wash over me that I hadn't felt earlier. I bathed in this loving energy for as long as possible, knowing that this loving energy had the power to heal me.

In other words, when I became 100% okay with my choice to call my father, it became a nonissue and I was okay with it. I once again knew that it was for the greater good and realized without a shadow of a doubt that my inner voice will never lead me astray. I recognized that its perspective is at least a thousand times greater than mine. This surrendering meditation allowed for me to continue to love my father unconditionally regardless of whether we'd ever speak again. I embodied love.

I realized that I'd likely caused myself to become a pariah, not just with my father, but also with my one brother and sister-in-law. My main focus was to be centred in self-love and staying expansive. I did feel regret at one point for not having had the courage to have this talk with my father years earlier, but I now know that I hadn't been ready. Back then I had still been functioning from fear and would never have considered rocking the boat like this. I did, however, dabble a little bit, by writing a blog about my father after my visit with him during the summer of 2018. I hadn't gone into much detail at all, but enough that my brother sent me a message suggesting that I take the blog down in case dad read it. I took it down, because I was not ready to face an angry father after all. Had he read that blog or had I told him everything back then, it would probably have been much worse. I did not love myself unconditionally at that time. It likely would have taken me for a tailspin. Everything happens in its own time.

In my opinion, self-love is the most important antidote for this situation, or any other situation for that matter.

A few weeks had passed when I received a message from my brother, Roelof, that our father wanted to talk to me, but wanted me to call him. I did. It was a strange phone call where he did not bring up the previous phone conversation at all, and I didn't either. I knew that my father never apologized. Perhaps he was giving me an opportunity to apologize? By this time I had managed to release all doubt and regret regarding the talk and knew that I had nothing to apologize for. The phone call was finished awkwardly while I told him that I loved him, something that he didn't reiterate, and we hung up. That was to be the last time that I spoke with him before he left this physical realm. My sister-in-law later informed me that he didn't want the other phone conversation to be the last one before he died, in case I may feel regret for the rest of my life. This wouldn't have been the case; however, I certainly appreciated this gesture.

My father was taken into the hospital about two months later with a broken hip. He left his body six days later with his two sons and daughter-in-law at his bedside. He did not want me there. Thanks to all the surrendering meditations, I was at peace with that.

CHAPTER 19

Work, Work, Work

"I can run circles around people half my age." This was my line and I used it quite often. And I proved it by working multiple jobs, keeping up a pretty intense exercise regime, and making sure that I was there for my kids and Ian as much as possible. Not many would have been able to keep this pace going, including myself...apparently. My body had given me lots of nudges that suggested it would be wise to slow down my pace; however, I turned a blind eye. Those nudges got stronger and stronger until I could no longer ignore them. I was face-to-face with a cancer diagnosis for the second time in ten years. One would think that I would have wisened up a bit after my first diagnosis, but the drive within me was relentless. I continued to muscle through life even after that first diagnosis.

Leading up to that first diagnosis, in the spring of 2007, I was working three jobs, all part-time mind you, but they added up to a lot of hours every week…too many hours. You would think that going through surgery, chemo, and radiation would have me taking a leave of absence from all of those jobs, but you would think wrong. I did take a leave from two of the jobs only because the oncologist was worried about exposure to germs. I continued working one of the jobs, the most demanding one of them all, but I could do a good chunk of this job from the comforts of my own home. I remember telling people that continuing to work was good for me, otherwise I'd just have too much time on my hands to think about my situation. Yup, I was the queen of avoidance.

Approximately seven months after getting diagnosed, I completed all the treatments and was told that I was cancer-free. Within days of my last radiation treatment, I was back to adding the other two jobs to my repertoire, teaching and serving. It was the beginning of December and Ian had made the suggestion that I take a break to rest my body and wait until after the Christmas holidays before going back to work. I would not hear of it. I had something to prove, and it was driving me to get back into the work force. I added a bandana to my uniform in order to cover up my bald head, and I was back to serving in the evenings during the very busy Christmas season, along with substitute teaching at the local schools.

My body gave out on New Year's Eve by way of a back

154

spasm like no other. It was the first of many back spasms that I had over the years. I felt paralyzed, both physically and with fear. It was a pretty effective way for my body to slow me down, wouldn't you agree? I spent several days lying on the couch, barely able to move, and filled with anxiety. Had the cancer gone into my bones? I went to the doctor and insisted on a bone scan. He tried to tell me that bone cancer was highly unlikely since I'd had a bone scan only a few months prior, but I wouldn't hear of it. My bones ended up being fine and I continued on with my insane schedule once my back healed.

I received a phone call from a principal of the local Catholic school a few months later, asking me to apply for a full-time teaching position. I remember telling him that not only was I not Catholic, I had also never read the Bible. He assured me that this was fine and that I would get all the support I needed throughout the year. I decided to accept this teaching position while still keeping one of my other part-time jobs. If that wasn't enough, I was also determined to prove to myself that I was 100% healthy by training for and completing a half marathon that fall. Good thing I was cute, because I sure wasn't very bright in those days.

As it turned out, I was far out of my comfort zone at the Catholic school. Accepting that job ended up being one of the worst decisions I had ever made. I was in over my head regarding the religion aspect of it, and despite the promises, the support was not there. Au contraire, I felt pretty ostracized, and thus, inadequate at that school. My body was vibrating to a point that my students would comment on it as I was writing on the blackboard with a shaking hand. Along with that, I was sleeping poorly and experiencing heart palpitations at night. I now realize that having been put through the cancer wringer the previous year had left me significantly weaker than I had been willing to admit, and this job was simply too much for me at this point in my life. The principal did not renew my contract for the following year, giving my position to a Catholic teacher instead. This turned out to be the best thing that could have happened to me, because if he had renewed it, I would have surely taken it.

Just days after school was out that summer, I was camping with my family. While sitting around the campfire one evening listening to Ian play his guitar, I took a huge breath. It was the first full breath that I had been able to take in months, and it felt like a thousand pounds had been lifted off my chest. I then looked at my hands and noticed that they were not trembling anymore. I realized that I hadn't been woken up with heart palpitations for the past couple of nights either. These realizations gave me a big a-ha moment...those symptoms had all been signs of stress. Wow! How had I not been aware of that before?

It was the first inkling I had that my way of living was not all that healthy. Sitting by that campfire, I made an important decision. I was going to slow down. I knew deep within my heart that if I kept up this pace I would surely be dead in no time. I made the decision not to go back to teaching.

Although I didn't ever return to the classroom again, my resolve to slow down didn't last. I was still very much driven by something beyond my comprehension at that time.

It would be another six years before I made the conscious choice to join the majority and work just one full-time job. Along with that, I also decided to listen to my body and quit jogging. Although I was still doing interval training, the bulk of my exercise would consist simply of walking my dog on the trails. Baby steps towards learning to relax more, even though it was still not in my subconscious makeup.

At one point, around 2014, I caught myself doing something that I had given my mother heck for years earlier. I was home alone, sitting in my chair having a cup of tea and relaxing, but the minute I heard my son come in the house, I jumped up out of my chair. God forbid if he caught me sitting and being lazy. It reminded me of a time when I was visiting my parents. My mother was relaxing with me on the couch with a cup of tea. The minute she saw my father drive up to the house, she jumped up and got busy. Like I said, I gave her heck and told her to sit down and relax. Here I had been behaving in the exact same way myself for many years, but on that particular day, a lightbulb came on and I was suddenly aware of it. I had mimicked my mother's behaviour.

From that point on, I forced myself to remain sitting regardless of who came through the door. Believe it or not, it was painful to do this for I was feeling so much guilt and judgment towards myself. I truly believed that I was being lazy. My son even made a comment about it at one point, saying that he noticed me sitting in my chair more, either reading or staring off into space. It was simply an observation on his part that didn't hold any judgment. Although I didn't admit to it at the time and kept outwardly calm, boy oh boy was I triggered on the inside! "He thinks I'm lazy! Everybody must think I'm lazy! I am lazy!" These were some of the harsh thoughts that went through my head. At that time, because I didn't know how to surrender to this, I stuffed down these thoughts and emotions and forced myself to continue to sit, figuring that eventually the guilt would subside. It didn't until I surrendered it years later.

When I had told Dr. Gabor Maté that I had continued to work while receiving cancer treatments, he asked me a question that changed my perception just a little. "If your mother, sister, best friend, or daughter was diagnosed with cancer, would you expect them to continue working?"

"Of course I wouldn't expect that of them" was my immediate answer.

"Then why do you expect it of yourself?"

Hmmmm. That kind of hit home for me. With that in mind, when I was diagnosed with cancer the second time in December of 2016, I made a point of going on medical leave and put my entire focus on healing my body. In fact, healing my body became my job that I took very seriously. I was so determined to heal my body before going back into the work force that I had to resign from my job a year into it, because they figured I was fit enough to work and wouldn't extend my medical leave. On top of that, I had to get a lawyer and fight my insurance company, because they also felt that I was fit enough to work. Goes to show how screwed up society really is. With those expectations, is it any wonder that stress is the number one killer?

Even though I had not been working for months, the feelings of guilt and the judgment of laziness were still firmly in place. With the help of The Journey, I came to the realization that I felt unworthy unless I was busy. My workaholic behaviour was, in fact, caused by a lack of self-worth, causing me to search for this worthiness outside of myself. Most societies promote busyness. People who work hard and long hours are often put on a pedestal and rewarded, no matter where they live in the world. On the flip side, relaxation is often seen as laziness. This is a pretty harsh judgment that I was encumbered with. The time had finally come where I was ready to surrender all of that. What a relief!

Ian is (thankfully) the complete opposite of me in so many ways. He's a good worker and he's also very good at relaxing. My father judged it as being lazy. It was this judgment that fuelled the discord between Ian and my father back in those days when he came to join us for the first Christmas break since my mother's passing. Ian was self-employed at the time with a tourism company. 9/11 had caused American tourists to be afraid to fly so they were no longer showing up in hordes to tour our beautiful country. Even though it happened a couple of years prior, the tourism industry had not quite yet recuperated. We adjusted, and Ian became the stay-at-home dad most of the time while I worked. Considering I was too restless to be a stay-at-home mom anyway, this was a perfect solution for us. My father disagreed. He firmly believed men should be the breadwinners.

Thinking back to that time made me realize that these harsh judgments that I was directing towards myself were likely intergenerational as well as a common trait in the Dutch culture. The Dutch are known to be a very driven bunch.

I skyped with Dr. Gabor Maté in May of 2019 when he, yet again, gave me something to think about. (That man is a genius in his field by the way.) I had told him that I was feeling restless and was ready to be driven again. To which he asked me if I thought that being driven was a good thing. "Well, yes. When I'm driven, I get stuff done." I told him.

"What is driving you when you're being driven?" he asked.

"Oh... hmmmm..." I pondered for a moment. "I guess being driven is not really a good thing then?" With that, the proverbial lightbulb came on yet again. I had been driven by fear. Fear of not being enough and fear of being unworthy, unless I was busy.

I also realized, had Ian been more driven, like my family and I, he would not have had the calming effect on me that he did, and that would have likely had even more of a disastrous effect on my health. Hallelujah for Ian!

Now that I had the awareness of needing to slow down, and I was in fact slowing down, all would be resolved, right? Not quite. I say not quite because I had slowed down significantly for a couple of years, and I still ended up with cancer again.

A few things were still needing to be cleared up. For one, I needed to surrender the belief that not being busy makes me lazy. And so, I did this surrending meditation.

I laid comfortably with my eyes closed and soft music playing into my head phones.

I set my intention: surrender the belief that not being busy makes me lazy.

I brought up all the emotions that were attached to this belief. I didn't hold back. I felt it thoroughly. I magnified it. As always, it was uncomfortable but I persevered. I allowed myself to feel the guilt, the despair, and the shame. I felt it all with gusto.

Then, I told myself over and over again, "IT'S OK that I feel guilt and despair when I'm not busy. IT'S OK that I feel guilt and despair when I'm not busy. IT'S OK that I feel guilt and despair when I'm not busy. IT'S OK. IT'S OK. IT'S OK." I said this over and over again until the guilt and despair was lifted out of me into the light of love. I knew when it was gone because I started to feel more relaxed in my body. I could breathe easier, and the knot in my stomach had disappeared. My throat no longer felt constricted. I felt a loving, compassionate gentleness wash over me that I hadn't felt earlier. I bathed in this loving energy for as long as possible, knowing that this loving energy had the power to heal me.

In other words, when I became 100% okay with me not being busy, it became a nonissue, and I was okay with it. This surrendering meditation allowed for me to let go of the belief that I had to be busy in order to prove my worthiness. Not only did I stop judging myself, I also stopped judging Ian for not being busy. Instead, I embodied love.

CHAPTER 20

Trusting My Inner Voice

For years, I assumed that others knew more than I did. Rather than risking failure (and yes, fear of failure was ever-present) by following my own guidance, I usually followed other people's advice with the assumption that I'd be better off. Actually, to be honest, I didn't even really know how to be guided by the voice of my inner being. The voice that I did hear on a daily basis in my head was loud and full of self-doubt. In fact, this annoying egoic inner voice must have been so loud that it overpowered the true inner voice that I'd heard others speak of, but certainly never heard within myself. Maybe this elusive true inner voice didn't even exist in me. Thankfully, I got confirmation that this was not the case.

It wasn't until my first Ayahuasca ceremony in 2013 that I got a taste of the empowering loving energy that resided within me. It was at that time that I realized I had access to this beautiful, gentle, wise inner being anytime I wanted. I also learned that this ever loving being always has my best interests at heart and has a much broader perspective on the going-ons of my life than my ego could ever imagine having. Tapping into this inner master instead of listening to the annoying inner chatter of my ego seemed like a great idea, but considering I wasn't going to have access to Ayahuasca on a daily basis, I had to find another way to get connected.

Meditation was the key to that amazing connection. Up until that retreat, I had dabbled a bit here and there with meditation. I liked the idea of it, but had decided that I sucked at it. Rarely did I last more than ten minutes before giving up. After being at the retreat for a few days, I thankfully changed my tune and embraced meditation. Much like committing to anything else, my meditation practice went through phases of total commitment to total abandonment over the coming years. However, as you've probably guessed by now, upon receiving the diagnosis of recurring breast cancer in 2016, I committed wholeheartedly to my meditation practice. I knew that this would be the most important aspect of my healing journey, which it most definitely has ended up being.

Up until now, I have only written about my surrendering meditation and as you have probably noticed, they were anything but quiet and serene to start off, although they do finish with a quiet mind, bathed in love and peace. I also practice the more common way of meditating where I sit with a quiet mind. These meditations made it possible for me to start hearing the voice of my inner being, the master who had the power to love me into tip-top shape. Once I started to be more aware of this voice in meditation, I started to hear it outside of meditation as well. All I had to do was listen, trust it, and I'd have it made in the shade. Seems simple enough. Still, so many times I have ignored it.

Even though I thankfully listened at the time when I received the diagnosis and refused Western medicine as a result, it appeared that I still had trust issues. Trusting in my inner wisdom was definitely lacking, and I'd learn the hard way that I was shooting myself in the foot every time I ignored it.

The last time that I ignored it was during the winter of 2018, when we were in Yelapa, Mexico on the beach. Against my better judgment, I went into the ocean one day while the waves were high and mighty. I was well aware of my little voice advising me against it, but playing in these massive waves looked like way too much fun. There was no way that I was missing out. In I went, and sure enough, within moments, my brand new, expensive prescription sunglasses were thrashed off my face never to be seen again. There were five of us that searched for them without any luck. Damn it! I should have listened. Enough already. At that moment, I made a deal with myself that no matter what, I was going to listen and learn to trust that inner voice.

Here are a few occasions where it definitely paid to listen.

As I mentioned earlier in this book, after leaving Yelapa, I headed to Europe by myself. Ian had made plans to go back to Canada where I would meet up with him later that summer. England was my first destination. I had not ever been to England and other than the weekend Journey course that I was scheduled to attend, I had not made any plans for the rest of the two weeks that I would be there. Believe me, I wanted to make some plans, but every time I meditated on it, the message that came through was not to pick any specific destinations, nor book any hotels. My inner voice told me to just relax and trust in the process. Yikes! Relax? I don't think so. In fact, it made me very uncomfortable. I hadn't quite mastered the trust the process to the point of being relaxed about it. It's a muscle that I will continue to hone for the rest of my days though.

Nevertheless, I followed the advice of my inner voice and showed up in England without a plan beyond the weekend course. It was the best thing I could have ever done. I had the most amazing time in England and I knew that it wasn't likely that any amount of planning would have given me that beautiful experience.

Having no plans pushed me way out of my comfort zone. On day two of the course, I was with a group of about fifty people who I had just met the previous day. I stood up in front of them after the evening activities and dared to put myself out there. I was feeling pretty jittery about it, but I went ahead with it anyway. After introducing myself to the group, I explained that I had made no plans for the duration of my stay in England and then asked, "Is there anyone who would like to go on an adventure with me and possibly be my tour guide?"

No sooner were the words out of my mouth, I heard from Daniel, "You can come home with us. We live in a beautiful little town near the sea." Wow. Could it be that easy?

Yes, and it got even better. The following day I was approached by another beautiful gal, Raj, who told me that she had a flat in Wimbledon, and I was welcome to stay there for as long as I needed. She wouldn't be there, but she'd be happy to give me the code to get in. Then, there were two other lovely gals, Lindsay and Catrin, who each offered to meet me in London on different days to tour me around. Catrin and I hit it off as soon as we met and had something in common. We both were healing our bodies from cancer. Lyndsay came from Brighton and met me in London. We had such a wonderful time playing tourists together that Lyndsay suggested I take the train and meet her in Brighton the next morning. She said something along the lines of "I have to show you my home town! It's so beautiful. You'll love it!" And she was right. Brighton was absolutely charming.

Quickly and easily my accommodations were arranged, free of charge, and I had locals who were proud to show off their stomping grounds and give me a true taste of the British day-to-day life. To top it all off, there was a heat wave going through the country making everything look even brighter and more spectacular. Speaking of taste, those Brits sure have a taste for beer and no matter what time of day or day of the week it was, the pubs seemed to be packed. Although I wasn't tipping back any beers myself, I loved hanging out at the pubs. They had such a great vibe that felt unique to England.

Along with my new friends, the rest of the Brits were very friendly and helpful while I was touring their country. It is a country that is so incredibly rich with history that there were moments that I felt like I'd gone back in time - the Victorian time to be exact. All in all, trusting and surrendering to my inner voice resulted in gifting me the most memorable time in England. I am so grateful that I had the courage to allow myself to be guided, and I knew without a shadow of a doubt, that there was definitely no looking back. I decided this would be the way I would play the game of life from this point onward.

***

I've mentioned The Journey a few times in this book. Let me share with you the synchronicities that happened as well as the inner guidance that I followed, which had me rubbing elbows with The Journey family for an entire year.

Shortly after receiving my diagnosis in 2017, my friend dropped a book into my lap while we were sitting on the bleachers of our local high school, cheering on our boys' basketball team. This book took my healing journey to another level. It was Brandon Bays' book called <u>The Journey</u> where she writes about her experience of healing from a basketball-sized tumour without surgery. Now, that got my attention!

I read the entire book within a couple of days and felt inspired. As I told Ian about it, he asked me right away, "Does she teach her method?" I had already done my research and was disappointed that Brandon wasn't scheduled to come to North America that year. There were other people facilitating on her behalf, but if I was going to learn this method, I wanted to learn it straight from the horse's mouth. Since the only options in the near future were Australia, Europe, or Israel, I had put it out of my head. Ian, however, pursued it and presented me with information that showed a reasonably priced hotel in Prague that was just steps away from the venue, and reminded me that we probably had enough airmiles for a free ticket. And the rest, as they say, was history.

The weekend with Brandon in Prague was incredibly inspiring and left me wanting more including attending the advanced Journey retreats which were available, but too rich for my blood. Since I wasn't working, I put it out of my head. I went home and started exchanging online Journey sessions with people I had met in Prague.

Several months later I received an email from The Journey

organization offering applications for scholarships. I rarely enter my name in anything, but this time, I listened to my inner voice and went through the trouble of filling out the application. As fate would have it, the stars aligned and I was one of the lucky recipients of a scholarship. This scholarship got me to attend advanced Journey retreats and courses in England, the Netherlands, and Bali. These were retreats that I never would have attended if it hadn't been for the scholarship. Considering that these retreats played an intricate part in my healing journey, I am so grateful that yet again, I had listened to my inner voice and followed its guidance.

While in the Netherlands at a Journey retreat in June of 2018, I learned about a pilgrimage that The Journey was offering in India later that year. Since this particular retreat was not included in the scholarship package, as appealing as it was, I put it out of my head and did not sign up. Then, while attending the Journey retreat in Bali a few months later, I felt myself drawn to it again. This pilgrimage was to honour the teachings of Sri Ramana Maharishi, an Indian sage. What happened at the retreats in both the Netherlands and Bali was mind boggling. There were so many signs… enough signs for me to take notice and rethink my decision.

The first sign that showed up was earlier that year, before I had even taken any of the advanced Journey courses. I had started reading (but didn't complete) a free online book about the pilgrimage of this Indian sage, but the name didn't register immediately when I learned about the Journey Pilgrimage. I didn't make the connection until later.

The second sign came when a man gifted me a laminated picture of Sri Ramana when he'd learned that I had cancer. I was deeply touched by his gesture. Not recognizing Ramana's face nor who he was at that time, I thought nothing of the significance of it.

The third sign came to me when I was in meditation and felt like my body had died, but at the same time felt my spirit bouncing around quite freely. I actually told my roommate about how weird it had felt before we went for the evening session. It was at this session that Brandon first started talking about Sri Ramana. She told us the story of how he, as a teenager died in meditation while still feeling his spirit alive within his body. This prompted Sri Ramana to awaken and live the life of a sage. I remember looking at my roommate in awe at this synchronicity. What were the chances that I had also just felt like I'd died in my meditation?

And finally, the fourth sign came when Sri Ramana actually visited me in a dream. It was a brief visit where he just appeared without saying a word, but it was enough to get my wheels turning.

I was torn. This ten day pilgrimage was going to put a pretty big dent into our budget, but I just couldn't ignore all those signs. Ian, of course, could care less about the budget and encouraged me to go. After weighing the pros and cons, as well as remembering my promise to follow my inner guidance, I made the life changing decision to attend the retreat in December of 2018. Considering I was still reeling from the news that the cancer had spread, the retreat could not have come at a better time.

***

Another example of trusting my inner voice is this book. I'm pretty sure that I would not have bared as much as I have were it not for my inner being encouraging me to be vulnerable and specifically telling me to write about supposedly taboo topics such as my open marriage and my experience with theft. As uncomfortable as that initially made me feel, I surrendered to this guidance and trusted in the process.

There are many more examples that I could write about where I received seemingly small little messages that actually still had quite an impact. Like the time when I got the nudge to offer to pay for a guy's groceries at the supermarket when his card wouldn't work. Hours later, while sitting on the couch, I was feeling incredibly expansive and high on life. This experience had shifted something within me which raised my vibration to another dimension for several minutes. In this moment, I realized the gift that this young man had presented to me simply by accepting my offer. Or the time I got the message to pay for my father's birthday dinner. And, another time, when a simple message came to me after I'd been particularly restless and anxious about what my future career would look like now that I was healthy and back in Canada. When I put this question out there in my meditation, what came through loud and clear was "Lighten up! It's just a game." Imagine how different this world would be if we all lived by those wise words.

Of course my inner being doesn't just speak to me. There have been many occasions where I would get a nudge, often in the way of tingling sensations down my legs, or a feeling in my gut, or just simply a surge of joyous energy that would make me want to start skipping like a 10 year old. Whatever it was, I'd stop what I was doing and say to myself, "Hey, pay attention here. This is important."

If I haven't yet convinced you to give this a try, let me tell you that having my physical being in sync with my inner being really is the cherry on top of this thing we call life. For one, the inner being is always in the present moment and knows your higher path. When you feel good, you're on par with your inner being, which means that you then also have a knowing. Let your emotions be the guide to your knowing - the higher the frequency of the emotion, the better. In other words, when I'm in sync, it's a one of a kind collaboration that makes me feel great. It makes me wiser. I'm more balanced and my timing is better. Everything always works out for me and I'm in love with life. And ultimately, isn't that what we all want?

CHAPTER 21

Letting Go Of The 'Jayka' Identity

As a result of listening to my inner voice, in December of 2018, I attended an amazing, life-changing, ten day pilgrimage in India put on by The Journey. My intention for the whole retreat was to surrender.

Brandon Bays is a yogi for whom I have such great respect. She is a gift. The energetic space that she holds for these retreats is invigorating and healing. I had been struggling with adrenal fatigue for some time when I arrived, and knowing that these retreats consisted of long and intense days, I worried about being able to keep up. To my surprise, I had no trouble whatsoever throughout the ten days. However, I felt my energy deplete significantly the minute Brandon left the property at the end of the retreat. I didn't realize the connection at first, until someone pointed it out to me. I was amazed that Brandon was able to do that. I would have loved to have been her sidekick from that moment on.

The first couple of days were filled with walking the pilgrimage and visiting the site where Sri Ramana Maharishi had lived. On the third day, we started to pair up with different partners of this retreat. My first partner was a beautiful woman from Israel. We followed instructions and took the time to take each other through the Journey process. Although I've had some amazing experiences from these processes, this particular one was pretty uneventful for me. I don't even remember what it was about.

It was our conversation afterward that stood out for me. We were getting to know each other, and I told her a bit about my journey with cancer. After a while, she asked me a question that would set the tone for the rest of the week. "What if it's okay for you not to be strong?"

"What? Not be strong?" That stopped me in my tracks. I had never considered that. It triggered a lot of emotions and I started crying. It had never been an option for me to be anything other than strong. We're supposed to be strong, aren't we? That's what society expects of us anyway. I certainly had always expected it of myself. This question opened a door for me. The need to be strong had created a lot of stress in my body and it was time to let go of that ridiculous notion. It's okay not to be strong.

Funnily enough, it actually takes strength to acknowledge

that it's okay not to be strong, and allow vulnerability to come into play. Even now, as I write about this, I feel my body relaxing just a little at the thought of not always needing to be strong. This was one of the quickest and most effective surrendering processes I had ever done, and it's one that I'll never forget. I've actually asked this same question to a couple of people over the past few months, people who have very high expectations of themselves. The look I get when I ask that question says it all. It is indeed a common misconception to always feel like you need to be strong. It creates so much unnecessary pressure.

Every morning of the retreat started out with yoga on the lawn. It was a type of yoga like no other, and one that I had only ever experienced at the Journey retreats. This type of yoga was called e-yoga which focused primarily on releasing emotions from the body. The yoga instructor somehow intuitively knew exactly what was required on each particular day to prepare us. She had fifty of us releasing heavy emotions all at the same time through crying, screaming, shaking, and dancing simply by using specific moves with specific music. These yoga classes synchronized beautifully with the Journey sessions that followed. It really was something else.

During one of those yoga classes, I became really angry at my body for letting me down and allowing cancer to eat away at it. I was screaming, crying, stomping my feet, and shaking on my yoga mat with the end result being that I was perfectly prepped for a Journey process where I could further focus on surrendering that anger. It was a brilliant combination.

The following day, also during a yoga class, I was doing the yoga moves and seemingly out of nowhere, this strong feeling of guilt came up for having been so judgmental and harsh towards my body all those years. I had guilt because of the eating disorder, guilt for overexercising and overworking, and of course guilt for all the judgments that I had projected onto my sweet and beautiful body. The guilt had me weeping on my yoga mat with regret, mumbling "I am so sorry" over and over again. The Journey session that followed allowed me to rise above the guilt and surrender it. It was an incredibly special moment, because for the first time ever, I felt true unconditional love for my body. It was beautiful.

Something very unusual and totally unexpected also happened while I was at the retreat. It was an event that took my healing to a whole other level. About a week into the retreat, I woke myself and my roommate up with screams of terror. Not being one that gets nightmares coupled with forgetting the nightmare as soon as I woke up, I chalked it up to a one-off. Imagine my surprise when it happened again the next night. I once again woke up screaming in terror, but this time I remembered the nightmare.

It was wartime. I was in the woods being chased by a soldier and ended up being raped. It was terrifying, and I

177

felt the energy of my father in that dream, except it wasn't my father as I knew him to be. That's when I realized that it was likely a past life experience. Apparently, my father and I have tangoed in more than just this lifetime. Since it took quite some time for my body to settle down after the nightmare, I decided to do a type of breathwork that Brandon had taught us the previous day which can trigger the kundalini.

Kundalini is the life force energy that is incredibly healing. Within moments of doing the breathwork, I felt the kundalini activating within me. It was like electricity surging through my whole body and considering I had no concept of time, I have no idea how long it lasted, but it was surreal. It put me in an altered state where a lot of pent up energy was released out of my body. The pent up energy was not even the result of this lifetime, but a previous lifetime. I would have thought that I had enough to deal with, without dragging around the baggage of other lifetimes. But apparently, I didn't have a say in that. So, good riddance.

Might I just add that my colon had been very sluggish for a couple of years. When I got up after the breathwork, I went to the bathroom, and well... I don't think I need to explain it any further except that it appeared that there had been a significant amount of terror stuck in my colon. My roommate did a Journey process with me later that morning which confirmed that it was, in fact, a past lifetime memory that my body had stored. Again, good riddance!

When we first showed up at the retreat, we were asked to take on a different name, either a Sanskrit name (a list of beautiful Sanskrit names was handed out for us to choose from), or else a name that came to us in meditation. I would have loved to have picked a Sanskrit name. They were so beautiful. But within moments of meditating on it, the name Grace came up for me. Really? Grace is so common and I wanted a unique name. However, that was not to be. Grace it was. We were told that it would be a name that we would feel we could aspire to be. Well, that much was at least true for me. I wore a name tag with Grace on it for the entire retreat, and it became the name I answered to.

Towards the end of the first week of the retreat I started to feel very uncomfortable. I was floundering. I didn't know who I was anymore. I felt like I was losing my identity, and it was scary. Albert Einstein once said, "The word I is an optical illusion of consciousness". It seemed that 'I' was starting to see beyond my illusion of who 'I' really was. My ego was desperately grappling at my identity, but it was slipping away, slowly but surely. It freaked me (my ego-self) out a little. It was like I was standing in quicksand. When you've been a particular personality for five decades, you can get a little attached to it. My ego certainly was. Surrendering my identity was apparently on the docket.

I remember the exact moment when I had let go of my false identity. It was when I was all of a sudden feeling incredibly heightened ecstasy where I was floating around in a different dimension and feeling beautifully expansive.

After coming down from that high, my perception had done a complete 180. I had lost my false identity and couldn't be happier about it. This expansive feeling that I experienced was amazing and something that I don't ever want to lose touch with. I will do whatever it takes now to surrender anything that gets in the way and causes me to contract, no matter how uncomfortable it may be to my ego self, including writing this book.

As mentioned before, this pilgrimage retreat was to honour the great Indian sage, Ramana Maharshi. I later discovered that there's a recently published book called <u>Who Am I?</u> based on Ramana's teachings...coincidence? I think not.

Something else that I didn't realize until later was that the act of letting go of my name - Jayka - during the retreat was an incredible gift that set me up for success in letting go of the false identity that had been attached to the name Jayka. After the retreat was finished, I went out into the world where people knew me as Jayka and had to be very conscious to not get attached again to this false identity that had been part of Jayka for so long, but instead to keep Grace alive and well within me.

Letting go of my false identity continues to be a daily practice for me. The ego still tries to attach itself to the identity of Jayka. It tries to take on a perspective that aims to keep me small and so-called safe. To offset this, I meditate every day, tapping into Grace, the beautiful expansive awareness that I AM, and the LOVE identity that I AM. This practice automatically lets go of any attachments or resistance that I may have taken on in my day-to-day life for it cannot survive in the light of love.

CHAPTER 22

The F*<k#d Up Need For Perfection In This World

I'm pretty sure that by now you've figured out that I probably deserve an Academy Award for fooling every Tom, Dick, and Harry covering all my troubles up with a smile. That smile was a message to the world that everything is perfect in my life. "Nothing going on here!" Meanwhile, my inner world was a gong show at times, but no one needed to know that.

Most of the time, I was oblivious that I was even doing it. It was that entrained in me. It was a default program. If that program had a heading it would be, "Don't let people see how fucked up I really am. Keep the facade going at all cost!"

I performed this program brilliantly, hence the Academy

Award. Of course, it helped that I'd never really looked sick a day in my life. I could fool just about anyone during my bouts with cancer. In February of 2017, about two months after receiving my second cancer diagnosis, I got a little inkling that maybe it was time to put an end to this performance.

I was participating in a San Pedro plant medicine ceremony where I was face-to-face with an array of distraught feelings and fearful emotions that I had so skillfully swept under the rug and was unwilling to acknowledge. These emotions were tied to the cancer diagnosis. The thing with San Pedro is that it sees right through you and there's no escaping it.

After quite some time of acknowledging these unwanted feelings and emotions, the message that came through for me was to take a selfie where I was not smiling and then to post it on Facebook. As you can imagine, the acknowledgement of these emotions had not been a walk in the park. In fact, I was a blubbering mess. So, with my face red and puffy, my eyes bloodshot, and my hair looking like a rat's nest, I was to take a selfie and post it? Are you kidding me? And, I can't even smile? Talk about being kicked out of my comfort zone. But I did it, right then and there.

But that wasn't all. There was more. The message that followed was for me to also make the announcement on Facebook that I had been diagnosed with cancer. Up until then, I had avoided that like the plague. It had been two months since the diagnosis and although we had told our close friends and family, and knew that the news was spreading organically, I had not been able to, nor wanting to, share this news on social media for that would mean showing vulnerability. I had even gone as far as asking those whom we had told to abstain from mentioning it on social media. I don't think I need to reiterate my determination to heal my body. Therefore, I decided in that moment to follow the guidance of San Pedro, surrender my feelings of discomfort, and commit to sharing my bad news later that weekend when I was more clear minded.

I wrote the "I have cancer" post the very next day while I was waiting to board a plane to Vancouver. In Vancouver, I had a connecting flight to Victoria, my final destination, where I was going to visit my daughter, Jellina. Having had my phone on airplane mode for a couple of hours while sitting in the plane, I had no idea of the sheer volume of love that poured out from so many beautiful people who had responded to my post. It was only later, when I sat down at my gate at the Vancouver airport, that I opened up Facebook and saw well over a hundred messages. I was so overwhelmed by the love that I was showered with. All I could do was just sit there, silently crying, completely oblivious to the hustle and bustle around me at the airport.

I was so oblivious, in fact, that I almost missed my flight. Apparently everyone had boarded the plane while I continued to sit there in a daze. All of a sudden, I heard my name called over the intercom and I snapped out of my trance. The flight crew had already boarded the plane. I was looking into the kindest eyes of a woman who was wearing a safety vest and was obviously going above and beyond her call of duty to make sure that I got on this plane. Completely frazzled, I ran outside when I realized that I didn't even know what seat I was in. Running back inside to ask her, she gently replied, "It doesn't matter, dear. Sit anywhere. You're the last to get on this flight".

I later realized that I had made quite a few people uncomfortable by not posting about the cancer diagnosis for so long. People had heard through the grapevine that I had been diagnosed but didn't know how to approach me about it. This last Facebook post opened up that door for them and they were able to reach out and send me love and support.

You would think that this impactful experience would have set the tone for me from that moment onward but that wasn't the case for at least a couple more years. Showing vulnerability was apparently not in my DNA just yet. Instead, I was constantly reassuring people (with a big smile) that I was doing great and not to worry about me. I even remember telling Ian how well I was doing, because I had barely cried throughout the entire first year of the diagnosis. Imagine. I thought that this was a good sign! That's how deep I was in this game of denial. It's also a great indication of how far I've come.

This wasn't the only area I strived for perfection in my life.

I had the same struggle and denial regarding my physical appearance. Having the perfect body meant that I was lovable. It triggered the bulimia followed by the incessantly controlled focus on healthy eating and my exercise regime. As we all know, the media has distorted the image of a healthy and acceptable body over the years causing an incredible amount of harm to our impressionable population. Women should be slim, but defined. Men should be muscled and strong. Anything that doesn't remotely come close to that is not acceptable in the eyes of society, and the self-abuse that has evolved from this is heartbreaking.

My very first Ayahuasca retreat in Mexico with Dr. Gabor Maté opened my eyes. I was the only person who was there to heal from physical illness related stress, while the rest of the group were all struggling with a variety of addictions. Listening to the stories of the other participants, I realized very quickly at that time that despite not struggling from a mental illness or addiction, I had more in common with them than I would ever have imagined. I remember feeling compassion for the addicts to a degree that I had not felt before. They truly were a product of their outer environment which created a lot of turmoil in their inner environment.

I've since come to the conclusion that the reason I could relate to them so well is because I too was struggling with mental health issues and addictive behaviour patterns. I've realized that the quest to perfection can easily turn into an addiction. If we are not conscious of the innate perfection that all of us are at the core, then we are likely to search for that outside of ourselves.

Along with my addictive perfection-seeking relationship with food and exercise, clothes also played a role for me, to a lesser extent though. Just this week I decided to finally wear a pair of shoes that I bought two months ago. I call these shoes my clown shoes for they are purple and make my already big feet look at least three sizes bigger. I bought them because they are good quality, water proof, comfortable shoes, and they were half price. There's a reason they were discounted. They are hideous! Even my friend commented on how ugly they were. So I had not worn them until three days ago when I put them on with an attitude of "these shoes do not define me and who cares what people think!"

They are truly so ugly that they're almost cute, and it made me giggle as I walked along the water that first day. I wore them again yesterday. Today, I even dared to wear them in town and no one even asked me what clown school I attended. I realize that choosing to wear these shoes seems really kind of silly and insignificant; however, when we start to become aware of all the seemingly unimportant little tidbits of our lives and tweak them consciously, while centred in love, it can add up to be life altering and have the possibility of creating the tipping point to consciousness.

But I digress…back to the similarities I had with those

struggling with addictions. I may not have turned to drugs, but I found other addictive ways that worked for me and that was all in my quest of creating a perfect smiley image to the outer world in a rather OCD way, while sweeping all my troubles under the rug. Denial was my way of numbing the pain, because I was not prepared to deal with it.

I know that I use the phrase 'sweeping it under the rug' quite a bit. What does that even mean? To me, it means that I essentially hid those troubles from my conscious awareness. I was in denial. Unfortunately, that didn't mean that the troubles had magically disappeared. Instead, my subconscious (the place under the rug) hung on to the energy of these troubles with a vengeance in the way of cellular memory. This eventually created dis-ease in my body. In other words, the pressure of my subconscious created so much stress in my body that it contributed to the cancer diagnosis. I could have just as easily pointed my addictive and avoidance tendencies towards drugs to numb the pain, but I'm thankful I didn't.

We now know that addictions to substances are often formed because they numb the unbearable pain that addicts often live with. What seems so unfair for the troubled people who have the illness of addictive substance abuse is that they are often shunned by society while people like me, who contract an illness such as cancer, are embraced and offered help. My time at that retreat forever changed my perception of my fellow human beings. It reminded me not to judge them for I have not walked a mile in their shoes. For that reminder I am grateful.

Having now surrendered this addictive behaviour of seeking perfection, I am filled with nothing but love and compassion toward my old self. Is it any wonder that I behaved in this way considering the perfection-obsessed world that we live in? When I look around, whether it be here or anywhere else in the world, I see a lot of people chasing this very sick idea that they need to be perfect in order to fit in and be accepted by society, whether it is by keeping a perfect household, a perfect physical image, a perfect work image, a perfect family image, or whatever else people feel the pressure of in order to keep up with the Jones'. Quite often, we juggle for perfection in most, if not all those areas, at the same time. Talk about stressful.

The irony is that we all believe that everyone else has their shit together and that we're the only ones who are secretly on this loser island of imperfection. Then, we beat ourselves up for not being able to obtain the unobtainable. Here's the clincher: we judge ourselves most of all, and put more pressure on ourselves than anyone else does... for the others are likely too self-absorbed about keeping the perfection game going in their lives that they're barely aware of anyone else faltering unless it's blatant. Do you see how fucked up this really is? And we wonder why anxiety and depression have skyrocketed over the years.

If you feel that you don't fit into this category of perfection seekers, you might be right. However, I would encourage you to put that to the test with the exercise below.

Ask someone who knows you well of their opinion of you regarding perfection and which area of your life is seemingly always to a certain high standard. Let's say it's body image and the way you are always perfectly dressed.

I challenge you to now go out to the mall or grocery store looking unkept and frumpy. Pay attention to your feelings and behaviour while you're out in public amongst other people. Are you feeling self conscious? Unimportant? Are you trying to hide yourself? Are you rushing through to get the heck out of Dodge before a friend spots you? If so, you have attached your self-worth to your perfect physical image.

You could do the same if you're a neat freak, by purposely leaving your home messy and inviting people over (preferably not close friends). How do you feel? Are you making excuses? Do you feel self-conscious?

These kinds of activities and questions create awareness within us. Awareness of our limiting beliefs is the first step of the healing journey, because you cannot change what you are not aware of.

You can follow this exercise up with asking yourself, "Who am I when I'm not perfectly dressed?" and notice what it triggers. Or "Who am I if I don't have a clean house?" and notice what that triggers.

For me, the answer to these kinds of questions usually involved fear of rejection. What is it for you?

You may have triggered some of your limiting beliefs. If so, you can follow it up with a surrendering meditation. Allow yourself to feel the discomforts and judgments fully while repeatedly telling yourself that it's okay to feel these emotions. Do this until your emotions have neutralized and there's no energetic charge to this limiting belief anymore. Then, allow the love to bathe you with the knowing that you are worthy regardless of what you look like or what you do.

Of course there's nothing wrong with dressing smartly or having a clean home, just like there's nothing wrong with me smiling, as long as it comes from self-love. If it's used to cover up something, or a futile attempt at maintaining control, not to mention keeping up the appearances of perfection, then it's considered a fear-based reaction. When you factor in that there is no such thing as perfection anyway, you can surrender the need, give yourself a break, and relax already.

My journey of leaving perfection in the dust has ironically made me smile more. But today, this smile is more relaxed and genuine and not covering up a minefield of kibbles and bits.

CHAPTER 23

The Bug On The Wall

As I was healing from cancer over the past year, and looking at life with a much improved perspective of myself, I started to be more at peace and calmer with a vibe filled with nurturing love. At least that's how I felt when I wasn't in the throes of surrendering. For a while, I was definitely feeling like I had multiple personalities. I would go from absolute peace to being a blubbering mess to being red hot with anger, sometimes in the span of an afternoon. The even keel personality that I'd put out there in the world was long gone. Talk about being unpredictable. This is just another thing I choose to surrender. Considering I've covered a fair bit of my "surrendering personality", I'd now like to explore the calmer, more peaceful personality that is part of my expansive existence.

Back in 2007, when I was initially diagnosed with cancer,

I experienced a sensation that was foreign to me, and therefore, I did not quite understand it. I spent a significant amount of time outside my body. I used to tell people that I felt like I was a bug on the wall, not anything as poetic and elegant as a bird in the sky. No, I definitely felt like a bug on a wall. Perhaps, this was a representation of how small and insignificant I felt at a subconscious level.

I blamed this sensation on the powerful chemo drugs. "These are some wild and crazy drugs!" I'd say with a chuckle. I now know that I was leaving my body on a regular basis. It was yet another survival technique, but this one was really cool!

While I was up on that wall nothing really bothered me. I just hung out and watched my life as if it was a movie. It was quite surreal and very peaceful. It really helped me get through my first ordeal with cancer; however, it also prevented me from going deep into the cellular memory and healing at an emotional level. Unfortunately, despite the Western treatments, my body did not heal at the core.

As I mentioned in an earlier chapter, I continued working throughout my treatments. My job was that of an event coordinator. I just recently learned that this profession has been rated as one of the most stressful jobs out there, only topped by the military, police, firefighters and airline pilots. Who knew? I suppose I should have, because my job stressed me out. The main event that I coordinated was a two-day mountain bike tour where there would be approximately 300 cyclists counting on me to have a fantastic weekend, as well as 100 volunteers that I was counting on to show up and do their job. Factor in the crazy Canadian weather, the conditions of the trails, sponsors, porta potties, and the insane appetites of the cyclists, and you have a recipe for many sleepless nights prior to the event. That is until I began seeing the world from the wall. Hanging out like a bug on the wall turned out to be a silver lining that lasted for the duration of my employment as an event coordinator.

My perspective from the wall was that the mountain bike tour event or any other event that I organized for that matter, was just an itsy bitsy part of the large scope of my life. I decided that it was not worth getting stressed over. There are many moving parts within the two day bike tour and I did my absolute best to dot all the i's and cross all the t's prior to the event. Then, and this is the key component (drum roll, please....) I trusted, let me repeat that, I trusted that if shit hit the fan, I would be able to deal with it in the moment, or find someone that could. I slept like a baby leading up to the event that year and it went off without a hitch.

As a matter of fact, I was much more relaxed throughout the weekend than any previous year and able to enjoy myself and really connect with the cyclists and volunteers. It was a revelation! Trusting that when I was prepared to the best of my ability, everything would fall into place. I didn't need to stress out anymore about the bike tour or any other event. And for the most part, I was a calm, cool, and collected event coordinator for many years to come.

My view from the wall lasted throughout my year of treatments and as soon as I finished the last treatment and went full force back to working all three jobs, I came tumbling down from that proverbial wall. Again, this confirmed my notion that it was just a cool side effect from the drugs.

Now, you would think that this revelation to trust in myself and trust the process would leak into other areas of my life in the years to come, but you would think wrong. If only... Nope, unfortunately that lightbulb did not turn on for me at that time. After my year of hanging out on the wall, I went right back to my old trusty and familiar behaviour of stressing out in all other areas of my life instead of just trusting in the process.

Thankfully, I did eventually incorporate the 'in the larger scope of my life' tool into a couple of areas of my life, but it took a few years. To this day, if I'm feeling stuck and indecisive, I will ask myself this question: "In the larger scope of my life, how important is this?" I will sit with that question in meditation. The answer may not come to me right away, but eventually I get the nudge needed to make my decision. Often, it also reduces my level of worrying - something that I was a pro at...just ask my family.

Years later, I suddenly found myself back on that

proverbial wall again. "How could that be?" I wondered. "I'm not on any chemo drugs." And that's when I realized that I could leave my body at will. I started to be able to do it on demand. If I felt stressed, I'd sweep it all under the proverbial rug, expand my energy out and feel the love of the Universe, up there on the wall. Life was great. It was very calming, but it was also a very effective way for me to play my avoidance game to the max. It certainly did not heal my body.

With that awareness I made a decision to stay put in my body and be with the issues at hand instead of sweeping them under the rug. There was just one problem. It felt heavy...very heavy to me, but I may have mentioned once or twice before that I was determined to heal my body, so whatever it took, I would do. I started having my doubts though realizing that healing should feel lighter.

When I randomly heard Dr. Joe Dispenza (Dr. Joe) talk about how it's much harder and more time consuming to heal matter with matter instead of going out into the quantum field to heal our body, I sat up a little straighter and took note. I then learned that I had the ability to change the cancer pattern in my energy field. By changing it in my field, I would then change it in matter, aka my body. (If I have just royally confused you, my apologies and may I suggest that you research Dr. Joe Dispenza. The internet is a fantastic resource of his brilliance).

The gist of it is that my healing journey truly was an

exercise of trial and error, and I was ready to give this a try. I already knew how to hang out in the quantum field (formerly known to me as the wall). I could resume my practice, but in a much more refined fashion. It was at this time that I started to follow Dr. Joe's teachings and meditations and learned that with the right intentions and level of vibration, miracles are possible in the quantum field.

This was pivotal information for me. I incorporated leaving my body into my surrendering meditations and coupled it with strong intentions. I also made sure that I no longer swept anything under the rug, but instead acknowledged the emotions at hand, surrendered them, and followed it up by going out into the field with the raised vibration.

Let's get back to the 'larger scope of life' tool for a second. Writing this book is probably the most recent example I can give you in regard to trusting the process and knowing that in the larger scope of my life, this is the most beneficial decision for me at this time.

Before I continue, I have to tell you that my motives for writing and publishing this book are completely selfish, where I am honouring myself wholeheartedly. I'm writing this book for me. And I'm publishing it for me. It's part of my healing journey. There is therapeutic value in the sharing of one's experiences, whether they be so-called good or bad experiences. Secrets carry a repressed energy and since I'm all about living an expansive existence in this moment in time, the secrets had to be let out of the bag. If anyone else reading this book gets anything out of it and breaks open to let the light in, then that's an extra bonus. But the main purpose of writing this book is, as I mentioned earlier, to follow the guidance of my inner wisdom and heal my body, mind, and soul. Regardless, this book will hit the shelves and undoubtedly cause a bit of a ripple in my circle of people. Therefore, I will continue to remind myself to use the 'larger scope of life' tool, so that it can keep me in a state of peace and focused on what's important.

For quite some time I have sat with this notion of being rejected by my circle of people and possibly ridiculed by them as well. After all, fear of rejection has been ever present in my life and caused a lot of heartache for me, along with questionable behavioural patterns on my part. It certainly was the root of all my people pleasing shenanigans. Isn't it interesting as I'm just now seeing this connection between the role that rejection has played in my life and how my willingness to write and publish this book is showing me that I truly have healed from that fearful thought pattern of rejection. I am willing to show my authenticity by coming clean in a raw and real manner.

I know I've grown leaps and bounds over the past year and I'm really quite proud of myself in that regard. At the beginning of writing this book, when the messages started to pour into my meditations encouraging me to write in a raw and real fashion and include my secrets in the book, I started to feel very uncomfortable. The people pleaser in me was threatening to make an appearance, sabotage the task at hand, and not go through with it.

I decided to do a Journey process on it, asking in that process for the courage it would take to write this book in the most authentic way. That process shifted something within me. It really made me realize that I am no longer that woman who I'm writing about, giving me a different perspective. I'm now writing it from the perspective of that beautiful bug on the wall, aka the quantum field, where my higher self resides and where the vibe is peaceful, forgiving, compassionate, and filled with love. I love myself enough to write and publish this book.

I also truly believe that there will be lots of wonderful people who will continue to love me despite this book or maybe even more because of this book. They will be open-minded enough and stick around. They will possibly see themselves in parts of my story and be willing to dissect their own story. No matter how it plays out, from my elevated perspective, this will just be a ripple in the river that may shake things up a little at first but eventually smooth out. In the larger scope of life, I trust that I'll come out at the other end a happier and more evolved human being, centred in love.

CHAPTER 24

If I Had A Penny for Every Time I Was Told To Slow Down

"This doesn't need to be finished tomorrow, eh?" This was Ian's statement more so than a question. Several years ago we started the huge project of renovating our home. It was a project that we did mostly by ourselves with the exception of a couple of friends coming over to help us here and there. Ian knew me well. I had one speed and didn't know how to shift it into another gear. The kicker? I never thought that this was a problem. I got shit done. That's a good thing right? Ian would just shake his head at me. He had a completely different perspective. Of course, this wasn't the first time, or the last, that I would go full force. Most often though, Ian didn't even have to say anything. He would just give me the look, and I knew this look well. But, it didn't slow me down because I just did not see it as a problem.

To this day, I have a buggered up thumbnail that is a reminder of the time when I spent six weeks scraping, sanding, cleaning, and applying two coats of paint to our huge fence. I was out there every day after work plus weekends too. It was exhausting, but I was driven and got it done. The neighbours were even commenting on my tenacity. For years, I saw this tenacity as a great quality that came natural to me, but in the end, it did not serve me well at all. It pains me to say this, but I probably should have listened a little more to Ian's advice. Maybe just that one time he was right.

Always pushing myself to do more was yet another way that I played the avoidance game. Along with that, it made me feel more accomplished and worthy. My ego played a huge role in this behaviour pattern as I would often brag about how much I had gotten done. I've already written an entire chapter on why I worked so much. This chapter is more about learning to listen to my body and slowing down.

Before I go on about the benefits of slowing down, I just want to quickly remind you of one time where my limited belief and behaviour actually created more for me, a lot more. Nothing is 100% bad. There are always silver linings in everything. You just have to look for them. Remember when I mentioned the time when I decided that I wasn't busy enough at work, even though I was, and decided that

I was going to organize an extra fundraising event? Well, I put the search out there for a keynote speaker. That's how I came across Dr. Gabor Maté's book, and the rest, as they say, is history. That time, the Universe gave me exactly what I needed, using my own predictable behaviours to get it to me.

It's funny how the Universe gives us exactly what we require. In the summer of 2019, I was housesitting at various homes where the dogs were all around fifteen years old. They're big dogs, too. What are the chances? I took Tucker, the senior golden retriever, for our first walk and quickly realized that looking after older dogs might be the Universe's very sneaky way of ensuring that I do not take off on a run, because there's definitely no possibility of running or even power-walking for that matter, with Tucker on the leash. Not that I was contemplating running even a little, considering the energy level of my own body. As I mentioned before, the cancer and all the healing that has happened had exhausted my adrenals significantly.

Adrenal fatigue is definitely the Universe's way of hitting me over the head with a two-by-four. In the past, my body has been relentless in trying to tell me to SLOW DOWN. I say relentless because there were so many whispers along the way that I ignored. I can remember as far back as almost twenty years ago when I worked as a full-time server. I broke my foot by falling down the stairs because I was too distracted to pay attention to how many steps there were, completely missing the bottom three. What makes that even worse is that it was at my own home. I was distracted because I had been juggling a million things at the same time.

My doctor at the time even suggested that this may just be a sign for me to slow down. Did I listen? No! In fact, I did the exact opposite. Relaxing and allowing my foot to heal was apparently not an option. Not being able to work at my full-time job, but needing to pay the bills and keep myself busy, I got creative and decided to start a dayhome. I took in an extra four kids on top of my own two kids, giving me a total of six kids under the age of four. That kept me busy. After six weeks, the cast came off my foot and I was back to my serving job. Did I stop the dayhome? Of course not! Instead, I had just doubled the workload and had Ian chip in too. Yup, I may as well have been wearing a cape, for superhumans do not slow down…ever!

Now, with the adrenal fatigue, I've had to remove that particular cape, and that's ok, because I'm starting to get a different perspective of what being superhuman really entails.

At this present moment (summer of 2019), my energy level is probably still less than 50% than what it was back in its heyday, leaving me no choice but to continue to slow down. I hate slowing down. It has proven to be one of the tougher things for me to surrender. My mind tends to be at least ten steps ahead of my body, and with my body not cooperating to my high expectations, I'm just a little frustrated to say the least. My power walks have turned into strolls; my multi-tasking days have turned into single-tasking moments; and, my "I'm game for everything" has turned into "I think I'll sit this one out." Slowing down has cramped my style, but it has also given birth to a different style, a beautifully expansive style.

Speaking of cramping my style, our son John came to visit us in Thailand in January of 2019 for a whole month. He told us that visiting an elephant sanctuary was on the top of his list of things to do. Since Ian and I had gone to an elephant sanctuary in Malaysia a few months earlier, I knew that it would be amazing. But I also knew it would be physically more demanding than what my body was capable of doing at that time. I had to bow out. On top of that, visiting the sanctuary was quite costly so this factored in as well.

Ian and John were gone for most of the day while I stayed at the Airbnb. I remember feeling pretty sorry for myself, and then feeling frustrated about feeling sorry for myself. On top of that, I was angry at my body for letting me down yet again. Then, there were moments of regret where I had wished that I would have gone anyway. I was on a pretty tumultuous mental rollercoaster ride with no desire to get off anytime soon. Although, by the time Ian and John came back to the Airbnb later that day, I had pulled myself together, put a big smile on my face, and listened to the stories while looking at the beautiful pictures. When I asked John at the end of his vacation what had been his favourite thing about Thailand, his response was the elephants. It still makes me a little sad that I had to miss out, but at the same time I am proud of myself for listening to my body, something that I wouldn't have done even a year earlier. Even though I wasn't there, I now relish in the fact that John loved his time at the elephant sanctuary as much as he did.

That was then; this is now. I've come a long way over the past few months in realizing that it's definitely not doom and gloom in this slo-mo life of mine. In fact, it's quite the opposite. My strolls along the seaside of Vancouver Island have awarded me with many wildlife sightings. I'm enjoying the wonderful fragrance of the flowers more (yes, I now stop to smell the roses). I actually sit on the park benches now and enjoy the views that I probably would have been oblivious to before. Ok, that all sounded like I'm now living the life of a senior, so here's one that isn't too 'senior citizen-ish'... I can sit and focus long enough to write this book. That's a huge accomplishment for me.

This is what I've come to conclude from it all: when I lived my life in the fast lane, multitasking and zooming around, I was only focused on the end result. Now, I'm more in the moment, enjoying the ride. And, that is the biggest gift that I've been rewarded with, my state of consciousness. When I do embrace my current slo-mo life, which is more and more of the time, I am present and filled with a heightened awareness. I'm in a state of expansiveness and feeling the love.

Only a few months ago, I remember saying that I wished I could feel the expansiveness that I felt in meditation all day long. At that time, when I did a meditation, I would come out feeling incredible. However, this feeling wouldn't last. It's not that I would feel bad afterwards, but the incredible lightness just wasn't there for very long after my eyes opened. Of course, I made sure to put that wish out there as an intention, and slowly but surely, the open-eyed moments of enlightenment were lasting longer and longer for me where I was living in full awareness. I know that my life in slo-mo has contributed greatly to this, because I'm not mentally distracted by all the busyness of this, that, and the other. For that, I am eternally grateful.

The effects of slowing down have upped my creativity a few notches causing the writing of this book to happen quite effortlessly. Only a year ago I attempted to write a book that, if I had written it, would have ended up much different than this one. It never came to fruition, because I couldn't focus long enough and lost momentum very quickly. Writing the book this time has been an incredible journey for me which has created even more healing than I ever could have imagined. I have been dedicating many hours every day to writing and feeling inspired without exhausting myself. Being forced to slow down has allowed for a different person to grow inside of me - a calmer, more peaceful and aware person.

I am realizing though, that when I am finished this book, there'll likely be a time of vulnerability where my ego will possibly feel somewhat lost. This is when I need to be careful not to fall back into my old addictive, thrill-seeking, high energy patterns of attempting to fill the void with activities outside of myself. In other words, I don't want to seek out these thrills just for the sake of the thrill. Instead, my intent is to stay in slo-mo, be in full awareness, surrender these tendencies, and know my wholeness in and of itself. When something does eventually come along, then I'm in the right space to enjoy that.

I'll ride the wave for as long as it lasts while enjoying it fully and when the time comes that the book is complete, I will put the question out there, "What's next for me?" I will then surrender to whatever possibilities show up, instead of giving in to the egoic need to seek out other thrills. For surrendering the need to feel these thrills allows me to truly be me and expand, because I know that the expansion itself is the thrill.

CHAPTER 25

They Were All Lies

When I was thinking about what the content of this book would be, I initially thought that I wouldn't need to write about lying, because that hadn't really been something I'd done much of, other than the odd white lie. I know that there have been secrets, but no one ever suspected anything. Since I wasn't ever confronted about them, I was never forced to lie. To be honest with you, if someone had asked me whether or not I had an open marriage, or if I had ever stolen anything, or suffered from an eating disorder, I likely would have told the truth. In fact, there were a few friends of ours who knew of our open marriage.

Then, a realization stopped me in my tracks...I had done nothing but lie to myself! How did I not consider that? I lied to the one person who should matter the most to me, but sadly, didn't. I constantly told myself that I wasn't knowledgeable enough, skinny enough, smart enough, cool enough, fit enough, or lovable enough. To add insult to injury, these horrific lies were what created the cancer in my body. I don't use the word horrific lightly here. As I started to realize the truth of who I really was during my surrendering process, the lies that I told myself started to dissipate and were replaced with the truths of "I am enough" and "I am worthy."

Having covered the "I'm not skinny enough" and "I'm not fit enough" lies in previous chapters, I won't go into anymore details about them. But, here's another biggie that I haven't covered yet. Maybe you're familiar with it. It's the "I'm not smart enough" lie.

I have two beautiful children who are both blessed with high IQs. It made school incredibly easy for them, and also for Ian and me. We never had to worry about any school related stuff, academic or otherwise. Although I have a university degree, I was definitely not a whiz kid. School did not come easily to me and I remember often feeling less than around some of the smarter students. These students also sometimes had an air of "I'm better than you." Although I apparently agreed with them at a subconscious level, their attitude also rubbed me the wrong way.

Years later, as a mom, I made sure to tell both my kids right from the get-go, when their school smarts became obvious, that their IQ is a gift. I made sure they knew that their classmates were not less worthy just because their marks weren't as high and to treat them with respect. While these were wise words, deep down I did not apply them to my own life. My disempowering beliefs were so deeply ingrained that I continued to feel less than for not being smart enough.

This feeling was compounded after I finished the chemotherapy and radiation treatments at the end of 2007. Although I was never warned about this by the oncologists, chemotherapy had permanent effects on me to a point that I was convinced I had Alzheimer's well after the treatments were finished. People would say, "Remember? I told you about this." or "Are you coming to that?" and I would have no recollection whatsoever. It stressed me out in a big way, and as always, Ian was my comforter, reassuring me that if I had Alzheimer's, I likely wouldn't know that I had it.

He was right. I did not have Alzheimer's. However, I did some research and discovered that quite a few people who have had chemo struggled with their memory and attention span. These chemo effects could last up to ten years. Ten years?! That seemed like a lifetime to me. It's been twelve years now, and the symptoms are still there.

Thankfully, I've finally surrendered to them by no longer letting them upset me. Additionally, I've adapted in ways that sets me up for success. I currently have 725 notes on my iPhone and that's even with me constantly deleting the ones that I no longer need. After my children's frustration with me piqued years ago because I didn't remember certain things that they'd told me, I had to have a serious talk with them. I admitted to likely having adult onset ADD caused by the chemo treatments and that the reality of zoning out was a frustrating byproduct.

"Just because I'm in the room doesn't mean that I'm 'in' the room. Please make sure that you say my name, wait for me to look at you and acknowledge you before you tell me what you need to tell me" were my instructions to them. It wasn't perfect, however, it helped within my family.

Outside of my family however, I tried to cover it up. There were conversations that I was part of where I would realize afterwards that I didn't remember much of it. Then I'd beat myself up over it. I thought I was pretty good at hiding this from others until recently when a very dear friend and I had a heartfelt conversation. She told me that she felt that I wasn't always there for her and that I didn't always seem to be listening, which made her feel unheard. It hit me pretty hard when I realized that this symptom of mine had affected the depth of my relationship with those who were so dear to me. This friend is like a sister to me. I was grateful for her honesty and finally admitted to her something that I had tried to hide from everyone for years. "I zone out... a lot!"

Along with zoning out, as I mentioned before, my memory is interesting, to say the least. What I can remember for an entire week will all of a sudden be gone, filtered out somehow, only to make random appearances. I realize that everyone has a blank moment here and there, but this is not just here and there for me. It's a constant that kind of makes me giggle now.

I am currently housesitting where I get to look after four pets: a dog, a cat and two hamsters. The two hamsters just kind of hang out in their cages so other than feeding them and having had a search party for one of them who had escaped and was MIA for two whole days, I haven't interacted too much with them. The cat and dog have my full attention though and I love hanging out with them. The dog's name is Tucker, an easy name that I remember well enough, off and on. However, out of nowhere, the name will go off into left field, and I am left wracking my brain, going through my mental filing cabinet to see if I can locate this elusive name. Most often I have to look it up... (yes, it's written on my notepad). The cat's name is Idgie, not a common name in my 'filing cabinet', making it even more interesting for me to recall it. I think she's starting to get used to the name kitty though.

So as not to put all the blame on the chemo treatments, I have learned from the brilliant Dr. Joe, that stress causes the brain to be incoherent. This means that the different parts of the brain don't interact like they should. On top of that, something else to consider is that the increased secretion of the stress hormones can cause long term memory problems as well. As you can imagine, the cancer diagnosis skyrocketed my already high stress level back in 2007. Add to that the poisonous chemicals of the treatments and voilà, I was hit with a double whammy.

Even though this is still factoring into my current life, having surrendered to it means that I now own it. I am no longer embarrassed by it. As a matter of fact, I can imagine that I'm not the only one out there who zones out or is forgetful. And anyone who can relate...whether having had chemo or taking other powerful drugs for any type of illness, or who is so stressed that it has caused symptoms of zoning out and memory loss, I invite you to surrender any belittling disempowering lies that you may believe about yourself as a result. This symptom, or any symptom for that matter, does not define you. It's a lie. You are worthy, period.

Another lie that I told myself was that my opinion didn't matter. I would keep my mouth shut instead of speaking up for myself. Of course, the 'don't rock the boat' behaviour pattern factors in here as well. I didn't even realize that I was doing this until I was in a plant medicine ceremony in February of 2017. It was the same ceremony where I was encouraged to post that unsmiling picture of myself on Facebook and tell people about my cancer diagnosis.

During that ceremony, I was also highly encouraged to write a text to a friend who had done something the previous week that had upset me. Despite being upset, I hadn't said anything about it to her. I knew that this

text would not go over well and that any ties that I had
with her would be severed. I was right about that. What
had happened the previous week was that we had co-
facilitated a course. We were both able to provide training
of a particular modality and she suggested that we put on
a class together at her house. She said something along
the lines of "I'm sure you wouldn't mind some income
considering you haven't worked since the cancer diagnosis,
and I'd love to help you with that." I thought that this was
very kind of her and agreed to be her co-facilitator.

The training day turned out to be anything but pleasant.
The concept of co-facilitating was foreign to her and she
talked over me throughout the day. I also became aware
that one of the students was a close friend of hers who
needed one more training session in order to be certified,
with the catch that it had to be from someone other than
my friend. I started to get the feeling that I had been
taken advantage of. She didn't do this to be nice to me.
She used me so that her friend could get certified.

Her friend was quite rude to me as well, making me
wonder what she'd been told about me. To top it all off,
when the course was finished, I got paid about a quarter
of what was owed to me, something else that she hadn't
communicated to me previously. Considering that I
drove five hours to her home and back, the money barely
covered the fuel. I felt used and manipulated and had
I been aware of these details ahead of time, I definitely
would have declined. I brought it up in a text that I sent

her the day after the ceremony. It empowered me and made me realize that I needed to stand up for myself more than I had been.

I also now believe that my opinion does matter and if I ever choose to co-facilitate again, I'll definitely be initiating more communication of what the expectations are on both sides. And this is where the silver lining comes in, for it is these kinds of difficult experiences that make us wiser.

When these lies are deeply ingrained, a simple statement of "I am enough" isn't going to cut it. It is important to go deeper and get to the core of it, surrendering all that is there. If you're not entirely sure whether this relates to you, I invite you to become the witness of your thoughts, words, behaviours and reactions. If you get an inkling that there are some lies intertwined with your beliefs, be with that. Question that by asking yourself whether this is the absolute truth or not. Go into a surrendering meditation and be okay with the emotions that are attached to this belief. Repeat "it's okay" until you feel the strength of this lie dissipate. Bask in the energies of love and compassion. Now replace it with intentions of empowerment and worthiness, followed by reaching for the feelings of empowerment and worthiness as if you already were that, which of course you are.

If you can relate to this chapter, which I think we all can at some level, then the time has come my friends to show yourself a whole lot more respect than you have been, and sprinkle that respect with a healthy dose of self-love and compassion. Please do not underestimate the power of this and how it can literally make or break you. These lies had such a stronghold on me that it almost took my life.

I know that sounds dramatic but I have never been more passionate about a statement. These lies contracted my energy field so much that it created a haven for disease in my body. For you it may not just affect your health but also create havoc in your marriage or in other relationships or at work or with money. It can seep into every nook and cranny if you allow it. Please stop feeding it and love yourself enough to investigate this notion and learn to let it go in such a way that you will believe with every fibre of your being that you are enough.

It's highly doubtful that there's a person out there that is immune to these types of lies in one form or another; we are human after all. I believe that we can all benefit from surrendering and find true empowerment within us.

Even though I've only written about a couple of incidents where the lies impacted my behaviour, I could go on and on with other examples of how the lies I told myself have impacted my life. Thankfully, I am no longer that person who constantly tells herself lies. In this moment, I know myself to be enough. And this moment is all there is.

If there's a moment where I become aware of a lie creeping into my thoughts, I jump on it so fast that it won't have a chance to gain any ground. My awareness of them is my weapon that drops me right in the present moment again, dissolving the lie. I believe that there will come a time very soon where I'll be present in the moment to such an extent that there won't be any more lies sneaking their way into my thoughts.

CHAPTER 26

"Lighten Up! It's Just A Game."

"Lighten up! It's just a game." This statement came through for me during one of my meditations at the time when we had just arrived back in Canada and was feeling some anxiety about my future. Life is just a game... hmmm, definitely something to think about. This advice certainly takes a lot of the seriousness out of the perception that most of us have about life, doesn't it? If life is just a game, like one of those board games that I used to play, then who am I in that analogy?

One of my favourite board games as a kid was Monopoly. Even as a grown up, I have played it many times with my own children. By then, the game had become more sophisticated with little electronic banks instead of the paper money that we had to work with back in the dark ages of my childhood. But, the gist of the game remained the same.

Let's explore this gist along with the analogy a little further, shall we?

First and foremost, what is the purpose of playing Monopoly? Well, that's an easy one - to have fun, of course! Ok, let's go a little deeper. How about the rules of the game? There are rules that we can either abide by, change, make up as we go along, or ignore. Then, there are the opponents to consider. How many will there be? Is there equality among the players' capabilities? Does everyone start at the same time? Is everyone invited to play or just a select few? What do the dice represent? Opportunities? Challenges? Doom? Do you set a predetermined time for the game, or go until there's only one player still alive? Do you even want to play the game or have you been talked into it?

Now imagine you are the parent in the room but not actually a participant. Your kids are playing the game.

Are the kids all confident players? How do they interact with their opponents? Do they take risks and buy lots of properties or play it safe and hang onto their money? Do any of the kids promote trades or do some hang onto their properties for dear life? Are they generous or greedy? Do any of them overreact? Are they judgmental towards themselves or their opponents? Are they compassionate and kind or are they bossy throughout the game? Are they indecisive and easily swayed? Is there a kid that gets easily annoyed? Are all the kids trustworthy and do they trust their opponents, or do some of them cheat? Maybe a couple of the kids take the game too seriously. Is there a quitter in the group, or is everyone determined to finish the game? Is the winner a gracious winner or does he rub it in? Is there a sore loser in the group who gets angry? And finally, are they all having fun? Was there camaraderie and laughter throughout the game?

As a parent you feel unconditional love for all the players throughout the duration of this game, regardless of how they play or the outcome. Occasionally you may lovingly remind them to have fun but for the most part, you are just there as a supervisor.

Now imagine that the game is over. Do any of the kids build a house on one of their Monopoly properties? Do they take their Monopoly money to the corner store and use it to buy candy? No, of course not. They've put the game back in the box and put it away until the next time that they want to play. None of it was real - not the properties, not the taxes, not the amount of time they may have spent in jail or the amount of money they ended up with. Winning or losing doesn't even factor in. None of that matters in the end.

Now, remember the purpose of the game. What was the energy that each kid brought to the game, and how did that affect the purpose of the game? Do every one of the kids feel better for having played the game, regardless of who won or lost? Although it's not the end of the world if they didn't enjoy the game, it does kind of defeat the purpose of the game, doesn't it?

Your life is the game of Monopoly. Your ego is one of the kids playing the game. Your higher self is the loving parent of the kids. The witness of the game called life. Your purpose in life as a human is simply to experience the game and enjoy it.

Here's the question of a lifetime...How could your life improve if you lightened up and lived by the notion that life is just a game? What if you could change your perception and become the watcher of the game, centred in love, regardless of the events or outcome? I can hear you already, finding all kinds of excuses of why this isn't possible for you. There may be too many hardships to even consider it. But what if you were to consider it? What would have to change? Your first response might be that your situation would have to change which may not be an easy task, especially if that involves your past experiences or getting rid of family members or coworkers or neighbours or changing jobs or, or, or...

What if that had nothing to do with it? What if it was something entirely different? I'll give you a hint....Nelson Mandela was a prime example of it. He was locked up; yet he was at peace. If you haven't guessed it already, the magic ingredient for lightening up is surrendering your perception. Notice that I didn't say changing your perception, because that is still attaching yourself to a perception.

Perception is partially created by your beliefs. It's your ego's way of identifying with life, and just like the Monopoly game wasn't real, your perception isn't real either. It's just your filter. It's like a filing cabinet where there are different files for different situations. There could be a happy file, a scary file, an angry file, and a victim file. There could be a work file, a kids file, the list goes on and on.

What happens when we let go of our perceptions and ditch the files? Considering that the perceptions of our life create our reality, it would definitely become a game changer. What would be left over? The truth. You would see an event for what it is without attaching a perception to it. You would not be triggered, instead you would remain neutral and at peace with what is, regardless of what it is.

Because perceptions are based on past experiences, it is important that you not go into your memory bank, but stay present with whatever the moment brings. Don't add a story to it. Don't embellish it. Just be with it. As a side note, it is vital that you surrender in all areas of your life for you can not be present with an event if there is resistance. Surrendering releases resistance. When present with a situation, you'll find that you become the witness of it instead of getting caught up in it. This is how you stay in that peaceful loving place of neutrality.

It's quite common that people are successful at staying

neutral in some areas of their life, but then are miserably caught up in other areas of their life. Whatever the case may be for you, letting go of your perceptions in all areas of your life will bring peace of mind. If your life is over the top busy, neutralizing yourself doesn't necessarily mean that your life becomes less hectic. Being present to the energy of love and peace takes away the frantic energy of the hectic situation. Having said that though, being present may bring an awareness that much of what was keeping you busy in the first place was actually an avoidance strategy. Being present has the power to alleviate that and may also make you realize that much of what was keeping you busy isn't worth your while anymore.

Being present takes your ego out of the driver's seat. It's a common misconception that your ego is bad and needs to be destroyed. We all have an ego and it is a very useful tool that keeps our lives organized and safe. It's when we allow our egos to run the show that things can become constricted very quickly. The ego is fear-based, and therefore, decisions are made or avoided because of fear. Resisting the ego will only strengthen it. Surrendering by acknowledging and embracing the ego-based thoughts will bring it up to the light of consciousness, causing it to dissolve.

How do you go about this inner shift of being at peace and feeling joy no matter how the game of life unfolds? Surrender, of course.

Whether you're in the throes of a situation and you're overreacting, or you're reacting in a less dramatic way, purely out of habit, surrender the reaction. Reactions are our programmed behaviours. Reaction is the game that the ego plays. When we react, we are not present.

When I find myself reacting to anything, big or small, there are two options that I choose from, depending on the situation.

Option #1 - Purposely pushing yourself out of your reactionary comfort zone

This is a powerful way to throw your reactionary programs out the window and put your evolution on steroids.

Stop reacting as soon as you are aware of it.

Become very present as the witness of this reaction.

Choose the exact opposite of what your reaction is (yes, this can be very uncomfortable).

Become very aware of the discomfort and surrender it. "It's okay that I feel uncomfortable and I keep doing it anyway."

Option #2 - Surrendering the reaction and choosing to respond from neutrality

This is a powerful way to make an inspired decision instead

of a reactionary choice.

Stop reacting as soon as you're aware of it.

Surrender your reaction (without beating yourself up over it) by repeatedly telling yourself, "It's okay that I reacted this way. It's okay that I feel (fill in the blank)" until you feel yourself lightening up.

Once you are at peace with the event, you will be more objective with the situation and can choose the next step from a place of love, without your ego getting in the way. This is known as an inspired choice.

The more you make a practice of one or both of these options, the more it becomes a habit. Before you know it, you can maintain neutrality throughout most your day and be the witness of this game called life.

Chapter 27

Celebration Time

In August of 2019, I finished writing about 75% of this book. The writing had flowed quite effortlessly up until that point. Then, all of a sudden, a writer's block stopped me dead in my tracks. I decided to hire a coach who could possibly help me get my book finished and on the shelves. Instead of finishing the book, my coach, Zensho, suggested that it may be a good idea for me to become a coach myself. After all, I had learned so much about surrendering and healing my body, surely there were lots of people out there who would be willing to hire me to help them lead a more conscious and healthier life.

Up until that suggestion, I had it in my head that I was going to finish the book first, get it edited and published, and then start my business. I realize now that the book was actually a bit of a security blanket for me considering I felt a fair bit of discomfort around starting my own business. This was something else to surrender.

My coach suggested that if I started my business before finishing the book, I would be able to advertise my business through the book. Considering I was experiencing writer's block anyway, and despite my discomfort of becoming an entrepreneur, this seemed like a good idea. Along with that, my inner voice had informed me by then that I needed to take a break from writing, because I had yet to live the remaining chapters of the book. I made the choice to get the show on the road, so to speak, and start my coaching business. 'Inner Health Outer Wealth Coaching' was to be the name.

Shortly after that, my friend Kathy told me over a glass of wine that she had always wanted to host a podcast because she loved to tell stories. She proceeded to suggest that I should partner up with her and we could be co-hosts of our very own podcast. I had never considered hosting a podcast before, but the minute she mentioned it, I felt the excitement bubble up. I didn't have to think about it at all. I was in 100%! That was how "Two Pals in a Pod" came into being.

My life was definitely being kicked up a notch. I went from being unemployed for almost three years to now committing to both a coaching business, blogging, and a weekly podcast. I seemed to be living outside my comfort zone much of the time and that's exactly where I needed to be in order to continue growing. Bring it on!

Thankfully, my body had finally healed from adrenal fatigue and I was able to keep up with this new chapter of my life. Adrenal fatigue had humbled me, causing me to be incredibly grateful for this newfound level of energy.

As I was telling people about my brand new coaching business, they would inevitably ask for the website. I didn't have one. Even though Zensho told me that lots of coaches start up without a website, I wanted one.

Who to hire for this job was the next question. I googled it. I asked around. I posted it on social media. I received a few suggestions, none of which felt right to me. Then, a friend suggested that I do it myself. "Sign up to one of those build your own website businesses. It's easy. I've done it myself!" she said. Easy for her to say. She didn't know how technologically challenged I'd been my entire life. However, a mantra came into my head that I had used when I was inspired by other people who had healed themselves of cancer. "If they can do it, so can I!" This mantra got me to successfully create the website for my coaching business.

Feeling empowered by this accomplishment, I then also created a website for the podcast. Not only that, I even volunteered to be the behind the scenes techie for the podcast. I went from being technologically challenged to technologically savvy in a matter of a month or so... with a little help from YouTube tutorials. Imagine that? Me, building websites, taping and uploading podcast recordings while figuring out the ins and outs of how to get the podcast onto sites like Spotify and Apple Music? It was incredibly empowering, and it really built up my confidence and set me up to dive into the deep end of being an entrepreneur. "If they can do it, so can I" will continue be my mantra to keep me growing and learning.

Since it didn't take long before I realized that I needed more tools to help me become a successful entrepreneur, I signed myself up for an online coaching class where they teach tools for coaching, online marketing, getting and retaining clients, creating programs, etc. The more I learned, the more I realized I needed to learn.

But, the number one thing that I wanted to learn didn't come from a classroom. It was confidence as a coach. It was definitely a muscle that I needed to stretch a little more. Figuring that confidence comes with experience, I reached out to some friends and asked them if I could coach them in order to get some of that experience. Other than the time when my daughter was three and I coached her adorable little soccer team, I had never been a coach. I realized fairly quickly though that it came quite naturally to me and that I certainly had played the role of a coach for most of my adult life as a mom, a teacher, an events coordinator, and a client services coordinator.

Networking was another area that I wanted to dive into. I attended a three day conscious coaching business event in San Diego. One of the topics that was discussed was the importance of celebrating our successes. Ok, that's a good idea and something I could probably be better at. I tend to be so focused on future goals that I do forget to celebrate when I have made an achievement. Come to think of it, I had met several of my goals already just with getting myself set up as an entrepreneur and hadn't really taken the time to acknowledge them, let alone celebrate. I resolved to definitely fit celebrations into my work schedule from now on.

The seminar continued on, covering lots of different topics to do with conscious coaching, and I networked with some wonderful fellow entrepreneurs throughout the weekend. Then something very unexpected happened.

I was aware that there was a group of people going whale watching on the Monday following the event. I had the time to go but hesitated. I'd seen lots of whales before and although I always get excited when I see them, I didn't really want to spend any more money than I already had. After being asked, "Are you going whale watching?" a few different times, I realized how silly it was for me not to go. Resistance to spending money was a familiar reaction that showed me that I was allowing my fearful ego to be in the driver's seat. Not happening! I decided, "I'm rising above the ego, doing the opposite of my reaction and spending the money to go whale watching!"

On Sunday, I approached Ann, the whale watching organizing lady to let her know that I'd like to sign up.

"Great," she said. "There'll be a really good chance that we'll see a pod of dolphins too." No sooner were those words out of her mouth that I felt a lump rise up in my throat with tears welling up in my eyes. "What is going on?" I wondered aloud. "I'm getting emotional just at the mention of dolphins?" I had never seen dolphins in the wild but still...this was a bit much. Ann could see my emotional reaction and told me that dolphins are incredibly spiritual animals. She then proceeded to tell me that she runs a retreat in the Bahamas where people get to swim with wild dolphins every day for six days. Well, if that didn't get me going! Right into a full on, cleansing cry (aka the ugly cry)!

This just made no sense at all. Why was I falling apart like this? I don't exactly remember the conversation after except when Ann asked me, "Have you celebrated the fact that you've healed your body from cancer?" Bingo! She nailed it right on the head. Now I was a complete blubbering mess. Apparently she saw a connection between the dolphins and a lack of celebrating...not sure how she put two and two together. A sixth sense, perhaps?

The realization that came with all of this was that I had not really taken the time to celebrate my healing success.

February 18, 2019 is a day I will never forget. In fact, I remember it like it was yesterday. There I was, sitting in the doctor's office in Chang Mai, Thailand. "There are no active cancer cells in your body," the doctor says with a thick accent. *Wait! What? Did I hear him correctly?*

"Did you just say that there is no cancer in my body?" I ask him.

"Yes. You are cancer free."

"Just to clarify, there is no active cancer in my breast, my cervix, or my uterus?" I ask him with disbelief."

"No, you are cancer free."

Not even four months earlier I had been told that it had spread and now its gone? Just like that? The only thing I've been doing in that time was surrendering in meditation. Could that have actually healed me?

Tears of relief silently rolled down my cheeks as I sat there in shock. My greatest wish had come true and I had not seen it coming. I was cancer-free. Wow!

"You happy right?" the doctor asks me in broken English. I laugh through my tears.

"Yes! Of course I'm happy!"

The doctor proceeded to share the rest of the test results with me and sent me on my way. Thankfully, I was given all the documents of the results because none of what he said registered in my brain beyond the moment of being told that I was cancer-free. As you probably realize, getting this news did not mean that my healing journey was complete. I still had a lot more to surrender; however, this was the most surreal moment of triumph in my healing journey.

I walked outside towards Ian, who was waiting for me on the scooter and looked him in the eye with awe. "The results showed that there is no active cancer in my body." I told him.

"What?" he said.

"I'm cancer-free!" I reiterated.

The two of us stood in the parking lot, hugging and crying before we took off down the country road. The freedom I felt was incredible and I screamed with exuberance at the top of my lungs while sitting on the back of the scooter. I was grinning from ear to ear with the wind in my face and arms raised above my head while securely leaning into Ian. It was truly exhilarating.

Unfortunately, this celebration was doused significantly when I called my father the next day. I was so excited to share this news with him that I was a bit shocked that he didn't congratulate me. In fact, he didn't even acknowledge it. Did he not believe me? I remembered the reason why he didn't want to help me out financially a couple of years before. He didn't believe in my methods. Now that my methods had actually healed my body, was it possible that he wasn't able to acknowledge it, because that would mean that he would have to admit he was wrong? Not only that, most of my extended family also didn't acknowledge it. I allowed all of this to really put a damper on myself and alas, the celebration came to a screeching halt.

Yet another piece of the puzzle that I surrendered. I repeated the words, "It's okay to feel sad. It's okay that my healing wasn't acknowledged. It's okay."

To be fair, I'm fully aware that the concept of healing from cancer through surrendering and meditating is beyond the comprehension of most people, leaving them to doubt my success. Nevertheless, I allowed it to dampen my celebration while doubt started to creep in for me as well. Maybe the doctor had it all wrong. Thankfully there have been numerous times since then where I've had confirmation that I am indeed healed.

As the ever-loving witness, I take a moment again with the woman I was then, filled with doubt and sadness. I hug her energetically and tell her it's okay to feel the rejection and doubt. It's okay to feel hurt for not being acknowledged, understood, or believed as I embrace her with compassionate love. I encourage her to celebrate her vibrant health, every day of her life, wholeheartedly, regardless of how others perceive it.

Maybe this celebration will involve the magic of swimming with wild dolphins some day, who knows?

CHAPTER 28

Let's Recap

I just want to take this moment to say thank you for making it this far into the book. May I assume that you're also interested in surrendering your life in order to create a feeling of freedom that is out of this world? Then, congratulations are in order for being willing to explore your inner world and let go. Take a moment to celebrate your willingness right now! It takes courage to open up to the pain body.

There will likely be times that it becomes overwhelming for you. May I remind you to be compassionate, gentle, and loving with yourself when those moments arise.

What is a pain body? It's an accumulation of painful life experiences that we haven't yet surrendered, and therefore, are festering and wreaking havoc in our bodies. Sometimes

I refer to the pain body as a treasure, because when you open up to your inner treasure and surrender to it, what's left behind is a gem that is beyond magnificent. There are no words to describe what arises when you embody this gem, this love.

Your ego may retaliate with "Why would I send out a search party and look for trouble? My life's really not that bad." I would have agreed with you back in the day when I didn't think my life was all that bad either. Now I know it's a vital step to set the stage for your superstar self to finally come through. And let me tell you, there's a massive difference between living a life that's not too bad and knocking it out of the park!

About that search party: Where to start? How to look? What to use? So many questions.

First things first. Get rid of all the noise that's just distracting you, and start meditating. Before you even think about making excuses, and I know what's coming, let me just share this Zen saying with you:

> "You should meditate for 20 minutes every day. And if you don't have time, then you should meditate for one hour."

Even though I'm not a fan of the word *should* you get the drift, right? If this is not something you've ever done, I would highly recommend that you join a meditation class, either online or find one in your community. There is no right or wrong way to meditate. Let go of the worries that you're not doing it perfectly. Much like anything, it will take some time to hone the muscle and learn this vital skill. Please be patient with yourself and don't give up. If you can quiet your mind for just a couple of minutes, that's a great start. I know from experience that there are good days and not such good days with meditation, but there really are no bad. For me, the more difficult and frustrating meditations have had a greater impact, because they have given me the opportunity to dig in and persevere. This perseverance will go a long way.

There's not a human being on this planet who hasn't had some form of trauma at some point in their life and that includes you. Think about your childhood. It could be something as common as a parents' divorce, changing schools, losing a friend, being bullied, etc. Or maybe it happened more recently. Was there a bad break up? Did you get fired or let go from your last job? Or maybe you lost all your money in the stock market? Whatever it was for you, I'm telling you, it's worth looking into.

What if the effects of this are still festering in your body? You may be thinking, "But that happened decades ago. I've dealt with it. I've moved on." Maybe you have, but what if there are still some remnants of it wreaking havoc on your cells? Consider this a tune-up. Most of us take our cars for scheduled tune-ups on an annual basis. May I suggest that you give the same consideration to your most precious piece of machinery, your body?

Meditation is a way to quiet the mind while simultaneously witnessing and being okay with any thoughts and emotions that may arise. It's a way to get in touch with your body. It's a way to cultivate unconditional love towards yourself. In other words, it serves as a vehicle to being a truly loving person.

Let's get one thing straight. You don't need fixing. Yes, you read that right. There's nothing wrong with you. As a matter of fact, it's the notion that you need fixing that gets in the way of the best version of your life. It's time to acknowledge this and embrace all the intricate beautiful parts of you. Let me just say that again because it bears repeating. "There is nothing wrong with you. You are beautiful and whole just the way you are." It's the discovery and honouring of this wholeness, the gem that you are, that brings about the healing.

One more thing, please let go of any expectations when you dive into the deep end of your meditation practice. Yes, meditation can definitely get you into total bliss. However, it can also bring up all kinds of stuff that will trigger you and make you want to run for the hills. Those would be the times where you have just dug up a treasure that needs some tender loving care. The best thing to do is not run for the hills, but to stay. Stay with it without judgments, especially when you feel so uncomfortable that you're squirming in your seat. Stay with it for as long as it takes and trust that eventually something will shift within you. Loving compassion will arise eventually. Self-compassion is key in letting go of harmful patterns. As a matter of fact, without compassion, you will not be able to see the treasure for what it truly is.

You may find that your life becomes an emotional roller coaster once you start your meditation practice. I was beginning to think that I had multiple personality disorder at one point, and believe it or not, this is a good sign. This is simply an indication that you have become more aware and that you are no longer able to hide anything from yourself. It will eventually get easier to surrender as long as you continue to move towards the emotional pain body and stay with the emotions of your limiting belief for as long as it takes. That is what creates inner peace.

To recap: meditation isn't about getting it just right, or finding that ideal state. No, it's about staying present in the moment, whatever the moment brings, and embracing it with the energy of compassion.

I hope I've convinced you enough to give this a go. If so, let's do it.

First, let's set you up for success and take a moment to come up with your intention. This intention will be the road map for your meditation. It could be very general such as "Please show me what I need to be aware of in my emotional pain body." Or, if you already know which incident you want to dissect, your intention could be something like "I intend to become aware of the core emotions that are wreaking havoc in my thyroid." Or "How can I use this suffering as a vehicle for transformation?"

Here are some helpful tips on how to make your intentions have more oomph:

Take some time and write down your intention on a piece of paper. This plants the seed.

Ensure that your intention is written positively. For example, instead of "I don't want any more pain in my stomach," your intention could be "I intend to be with the pain and understand the root cause of the pain in my stomach."

Read your intention out loud before you start your meditation.

Let go of any expectations. This is an important step. Expectations often have an energy of desperation attached and that is definitely not something you want to send out into the Universe!

Believe in this process. Doubt will crash the party in a heartbeat.

And finally, be open to whatever comes your way. Remember, it often doesn't look anything like what you had envisioned.

With your intention set, you are now ready to start your surrendering meditation. Keep in mind that you may not have any a-ha moments during your first meditation, or second, or even third, but please don't fret. The more impatient you become, the longer it will take. Remember the Universe is all about the Law of Attraction. Impatience only brings about more reasons for you to become more impatient, kind of like beating your head against the wall. There's also the possibility that you won't even receive any clues during your meditations. They'll come to you when you least expect it, like when you're out walking your dog or you're sitting in traffic at a red light.

This brings me to my next point. BE AWARE of your thoughts at all times throughout the day. Become the watcher of your thoughts. This in and of itself will bring stillness into your life. Being the watcher takes your ego out of the driver's seat and places your consciousness front and centre. While you're at it, you may as well become the watcher of your behaviours, your emotions, and your conversations, too. In other words, put the magnifying glass on all of you so that you can figure out what makes you tick and what needs surrendering.

When you hit the jackpot of your pain body you will feel thoughts like, "Poor, poor me. Life was so unfair to me. Time for a pity party." Hang on! Hang on! Been there, done that, and got the t-shirt. This is not the route to superstardom! Victim energy is pretty low on the totem pole of vibrations, and there ain't no healin' happening down there! Let's get something straight right away. Life doesn't happen to you. It happens FOR you. In other words, take responsibility, surrender, and let it strengthen you to Wonder Woman and/or Superman proportions!

Not convinced yet? What if I told you that you as a soul had set up a contract with your ex before you even plopped your cute little ass into this world? What if I told you that you picked your parents with great care knowing that they would push your buttons in ways that would cause havoc in your life? What if I told you that the gist of your life was by design, setting yourself up for exponential growth? The tougher the situation, the more likely that you will break down and surrender to it. In other words, your soul is a pretty smart cookie and arranged for you to have people and events in your life that create the treasures within you to be exposed. It knew that hardship would provide a greater opportunity to direct you to that magnificent hidden gem that has always been the greater part of you. It's an unfortunate fact that we humans tend to evolve more rapidly when faced with adversity. Let's put a stop to that! Don't get me wrong. I'm all for evolution. However, my intention is that my growth happens with a heck of a lot more ease and joy from this moment onward.

We have come to the grand finale. You've become aware of your pain body which holds the gem that has the power to shoot you to the moon. You have taken responsibility for it and now it's time to open up the treasure and find the gem that is in plain sight. Contrary to what you may think, you are not going to kick it to the curb and stomp it to death. No, whatever has come to the surface has been part of you and needs to be acknowledged without judgment. Feel it to its fullest while being okay with it, and then allow the gentleness, compassion, and love to bring it up to the light so that it can dissolve. It is likely that you have been avoiding this particular part of you for years, and ironically, that which you've been avoiding is exactly what is needing the most tender loving care in order for you to lighten up.

Did I mention that you're going to feel vulnerable? Oh yes! Sometimes you have to get to a very vulnerable place where there's nothing but fear in order to ignite the power within, and it's scary as hell! So I suggest you get real comfy with vulnerability.

If anger for your ex has made an appearance, remember what I pointed out before. STAY WITH IT, and trust that compassion will eventually make an appearance. Feel the anger; let it grow within you; let it engulf you while allowing your body do what it does, whether it's sweating, shaking, crying, all of the above, or none of the above. Remember that there is no right or wrong here. When it has taken its course, and be patient for it could take a while, you'll feel your body calm down and relax. When this happens, allow the love to flow in, supercharging the love even more by opening your heart.

Opening up my heart was a vital part of my surrendering meditations, and just in case you're not quite sure what that means, let me explain it.

The heart is an incredibly powerful energy centre that is

associated with unconditional love, compassion, forgiveness, peace, and joy. Keep in mind that your thoughts are energy. Where you place your thoughts, your energy goes. The way that I open up this centre is by first placing my awareness in my heart. Then, I imagine that there are big barn doors (inner farm girl coming out here) that open up in front of the heart and I release all the beautiful heart energy. I supercharge the love and allow it to flow freely through my whole body and into my aura with the knowledge that it is a powerful healing energy. Next, I would just relax and bask in the energies of love, compassion, and joy for as long as possible. It's a lovely way to finish these tough meditations.

Consciously opening your heart and spreading love doesn't just have to be an exercise exclusive to your meditations. It's something that I do on many occasions throughout my day. Sometimes I do this with the intent of sending healing love to someone else, and sometimes it's for me. Either way, I know it benefits me, and it benefits everyone. After all, we are ONE.

May I suggest that you do it just for the heck of it. How many times will you remember to open up your heart in a day? This is a great exercise of being present.

As you continue to practice surrendering meditations, keep in mind that it can sometimes happen in stages. You may have released all of the emotion of a certain event, or not quite. If you feel yourself getting triggered and the emotion is making an encore presentation later on, whatever you do, do not ignore it. It's best to be with it right then and there in the same manner as before.

I've mentioned this before, but it bears repeating. It will get easier! The more you surrender, the easier it tends to be for you to let go. It's like exercising a muscle. As a matter of fact, there have been numerous times when I have become aware of a thought that's related to an old pattern and I surrender it without even really going into a meditation. I just become very present and still with it, watching it bubble up, staying with it until I'm ready to let it go, holding myself in a gentle, compassionate, loving embrace.

Fully embodying YOU, the greater part of you who knows without a shadow of a doubt that you are whole, no matter what the situation, is the key to the mother of all gifts - FREEDOM.

No matter what anyone says or does, no matter what you've done or avoided, you are whole and worthy. For years I was told to love myself. Of course, it is easier said than done. As I started to embrace and surrender all the heavy stuff, I got a clearer picture of who I truly was. Then, the self-love came naturally. In other words, my surrendering practice brought me myself in all my loving glory. I embodied the love that I have always been.

When we come into our state-of-the-art physical bodies, we are not here to prove our worthiness. It doesn't matter how hard we work, how fit we are, what our sexual preference is, or what people think about us. No, we come into this world already worthy. We come to live life fully and to enjoy it. But somewhere along the way we got lost and forgot who we were. It's time to remember that we came here to thrive and love. It's time to remember that we, in fact, are LOVE.

I am writing this book to teach through the clarity of my own example. I now know that I didn't come here to suffer. I came here to thrive, to have fun, and to feel joy. I'm writing this book because I know that it will cause expansion for me, and by association, for others, too.

AFTERWORD

My Final Words, For Now...

Well, there you have it. You made it to the end of this book. I thank you for that. I'm aware that there will be a few people that may not want to be associated with me as a result of the content of this book. Considering I have surrendered to the people pleaser in me, I have also surrendered to that notion. If you are one of them, I wish you well, and I mean that with all sincerity. We are all on our own journey. Mine includes this book, secrets and all. Yours is whatever you choose it to be, and I honour that.

Despite knowing that there will be some raised eyebrows I have continued on my path because I now see the bigger picture. The bigger picture is that of magnificent possibilities and growth. I could have continued to fool everyone. I was brilliant at it. I was the soccer mom. I was the mayor's wife. I was a teacher. I was a volunteer. I was respected for the most part in my community. However, I wasn't living my life authentically.

The beauty of our lives is that we can choose something different in every moment. I'm grateful that I chose to not just live, but thrive at this game called life!

I am grateful for both my parents. I am grateful for my mom being so gentle and loving, and for my dad triggering within me what was needing to be surrendered. Without the triggers, I may never have gotten to where I am today... free.

I am eternally grateful that cancer showed up at my doorstep to heal me from the inside out. I'm grateful that it snapped me out of the trance of dis-ease, and caused me to investigate the truth of who I am. This truth led me to me, choosing for me.

My advice for you is to go within, untangle yourself from the web that you've created over the years, and start choosing for you. This may not always be the easiest choice, but it's oh so important and likely life-altering. When we live authentically, that which comes through us is authentic. The Universe will thank you. I thank you for bringing peace and love to this world.

Namaste, Jayka

ABOUT THE AUTHOR

At the age of 38, Jayka Duncan received her first breast cancer diagnosis. After surgery, radiation, and chemotherapy the cancer went into remission. Ten years later, the cancer returned and metastasized to her cervix and uterus. Unwilling to go through the same round of treatment, she opted out of having surgery and chemotherapy and set forth on an inner journey of healing.

Following her intuition, she and her husband sold their home, became minimalists, and followed their dream of traveling the world. Fifteen months of traveling turned into a spiritual journey where Jayka learned that the act of surrendering had the power to heal her body. She spent many months honing this surrendering practice, which eventually rewarded her with a 100% cancer-free body and a love for herself, her body, and her life that she had never known.

As a result of her healing journey with cancer, Jayka has started her own coaching practice teaching others the power of surrender, become a blogger, and created a podcast. She is also a motivational speaker. Healed by Cancer is her first book.

She currently lives in Western Canada with her husband, Ian.

For more information on Jayka and her work, visit her:

Website: innerhealthouterwealthcoaching.com
Podcast: twopalsinapod.com
Facebook: facebook.com/innerhealthouterwealthcoaching

ACKNOWLEDGEMENTS

I have to start with thanking my wonderful, kind, and loving husband, Ian. When I was given the diagnoses of cancer, Ian was given the role as a caregiver, not an easy task at the best of times. Ian was my rock as I navigated through my beautiful, crazy, and challenging healing journey. Ian stood by me through thick and thin while believing in me even when I faltered. Nothing fazed Ian, even when I was getting weirder and weirder (by society's standards) telling him about my inner conversations with my higher self. Ian took it all in stride without a single judgment. Ian's unconditional love for me shines through his eyes and it still melts my heart. Ian, I am so incredibly grateful for you and I love you to the moon and back.

To my two beautiful kids, Jellina and John.
Thank you for choosing me as your mom. It's been quite a ride and I'm so glad that you are part of my 'monopoly game'. Thank you for loving me and embracing me, even after I told you my secrets. I love you both more than words can express.

To Dr. Gabor Maté
Who knew that the day I met Gabor would be the beginning of a life changing journey of self discovery that has led me to ultimate freedom. I am incredibly grateful for Gabor and his wisdom as well as introducing me to the

healing powers of Ayahuasca. My trust in Gabor is what gave me the courage to sit in ceremony which opened a door that gifted me a powerful connection with my soul. That connection is getting stronger every day. Thank you Gabor.

To Brandon Bays and The Journey family:
Thank you Brandon for all that you be in this world. You and The Journey family were an integral part of my healing journey of self discovery and surrendering. Being with like minded people kept me motivated to stay on my unconventional healing journey. You gave me that and so much more. Thank you.

Bill Little – Clearly Conscious Energetics
I'm forever grateful for having met Bill and Ann many years ago. The channeling sessions with Bill gave me an in depth vision of what is possible. The number one message that came through Bill was "there is a 100% chance that you can heal your body if you surrender to love". This message and many more along with the technology that they use were a vital part of my healing journey. Thank you Bill and Ann for being in this game with me.

I would also like to thank You, the reader of this book.

Made in the USA
Monee, IL
17 July 2020